LIFESTYLE BY NATURE

ONE WOMAN'S BREAK FROM THE UNHEALTHY HERD TO ROAM FOREVER HEALTHY IN NATURE'S LIFESTYLE CHANGE HERD

Betty Holston Smith, Ed.D.

AuthorHouse™
1663 Liberty Drive
Bloomington, IN 47403
www.authorhouse.com
Phone: 1 (800) 839-8640

Published by AuthorHouse 04/05/2019

ISBN: 978-1-5462-1621-6 (sc)
ISBN: 978-1-5462-1620-9 (e)

Library of Congress Control Number: 2017917120

Print information available on the last page.

Any people depicted in stock imagery provided by Dreamstime, LLC are models, and such images are being used for illustrative purposes only.

Butterfly Image by: Peri Coleman

Author's Photograph by Chris Chrisman

Certain stock imagery ©Dreamstime, LLC

This book is printed on acid-free paper.

Dedication

To nature's wisdom that guided my way.

To my late parents, whose words, such as the following, were ingrained deep inside of me and helped me stay the course: "Hard work is the only thing that really works" (Viola Holston) and
"With hard work, you can master anything that you put your mind to" (Joseph Holston, Sr.).

To my siblings, who found the way alongside me.

To my husband, whose endless support found the way.

To my daughter, at three years old helped me see the critical need for seeking the way.

To my grandsons, who are finding their way.

To my readers; may your reading permit you to find your way as you look through my eyes and back at yourself.

Acknowledgments

"I believe in God, only I spell it nature," said Frank Lloyd Wright. I acknowledge Wright for making public an acceptable way to show equivalent respect across all religions.

Looking back, I clearly see that nature guided my life, not only to take better care of myself, but also to share what I learned with all who would lend an ear. Nature constantly positioned me in the right places at the right times, to experience and learn things that set the foundation for my nature-guided lifestyle. As a result, I have experienced the world differently than most others. I give a resounding philosophical tribute to nature.

To my daughter Traci, my motivator—thank you. I believe that natural forces worked through your game of tag to shake me awake to the dangers of not taking pristine care of my body, mind, and spirit.

To my husband Wesley, my best friend—thank you. You have never failed to support my efforts, even when some ideas seemed "out of this world."

I also owe a huge debt of gratitude to my late parents, Joseph and Viola Holston, who parented in concert with the natural forces.

To my five siblings, who from the beginning, and throughout life, accompanied me on my walk down nature's path.

To my older sister Shirley, the organized one and my rock—thank you. You read endless drafts of this work over the five years that it took to complete it. You always made time to read, digest, question, and comment, and always in respectful ways that helped improve the manuscript.

To my next oldest sister Joseline, my constructive commenter—thank you. You helped shore up the manuscript with your heartfelt commentary about the importance of my living experiences in helping make my messages resonate more intensely with those readers who need them most.

To Tina, my younger sister, my cheerleader—thank you. You always knew I could do it, even when I wondered if I could. Your constant encouragement always seemed to come when needed most.

To my first younger brother Joe, my creative cloud observer—thank you. You modeled for us all respect and love for the beauty in all of nature. Your nature-driven lifestyle most mirrors my own. Your life was a constant reminder of the benefits of taking nature to heart, mind, and spirit.

To my late youngest brother, Samuel Donald—thank you. You were my kindhearted running partner. You encouraged me to run marathons in the first place as you nurtured me on those early morning twenty-plus-mile training runs— patiently running with me at my slower pace.

To Sharon, my sister-in-law, my most microscopic reviewer—thank you. You are the kind of support that most writers need. Your minute scrutiny from a reader's perspective uncovered a flaw in my writing that improved my work beyond belief. Your constructive comments cleared the way for readers to more clearly grasp one of the main ideas of the book.

To my daughter Traci and her husband Gregory—thank you. You gifted me with wonderful grandsons, Hunter and Dakota. They have so enriched my life from the very moment of their births. They have lived and continue to live the lifestyle by nature every moment that they have been and continue to be in my care. I acknowledge their contribution to my life and to my writing.

Without Dr. Gabe Mirkin's daily radio talk show so many years ago, which opened my eyes to lifestyle over diets and the critical role played by nutrition and movement, I never would have gotten on the path to my unbelievable medical textbook-defying health. He was and is so far beyond his time, and I am living proof of his genius.

To Carol and Allen. Carol, you and Allen were the first ones to see the worth and to take on my "yuck" ways of eating as your own. Thanks for having and keeping the "yuck" faith and passing it on to other family members.

To Danny and Katherine Dreyer—thank you. As developers of ChiRunning and ChiWalking, you are my ChiRunning and ChiWalking family. Because of your ChiRunning techniques, I have run in line with how the human body was designed by nature to run. This means that I continue to maximize my running energy and minimize running injury opportunities, even at nearly 80 years old.

I still run ultra-marathons, including up to six-day races. Thank you both for your endless support.

To my VivoBarefoot minimalist running shoes—thank you. You enhanced my running. I have worn you exclusively for more than eight years, totaling nearly 25,000 running and walking miles to date, on all kinds of terrain and in all kinds of weather. You are like any one of nature's wonders—allowing my running and walking feet to do what's natural. As a result, you caused me no foot blisters or leg muscle stiffness or soreness. My "feet and legs have become stronger and more stable than people thirty years younger", says my podiatrist. Your designer used the biomimicry approach to shoe design, which seeks sustainable solutions to human challenges based on nature's wisdom. Your designer emulated nature's time-tested foot performance patterns and designed a no-gimmicks, zero drop, sustainable "barefoot" running shoe void of cushioning, arch supports, or motion control. My landing feet feels the road as excellent body alignment and posture are promoted and supported. You are at home within my natural lifestyle.

To George and Marina Tarrico, my "always there for me" friends—thank you. Everyone should have friends like you. You are not family, but then again, you are family. You gave hours and hours of your vacation time to review and comment on early drafts. Your comments helped to smooth out those early bumps in the manuscript.

To Lily Birch, my tech supporter—thank you. You helped me realize my cover design by putting the pieces together electronically.

To Jen Dicky, my life's enthusiastic documentary producer who became like my fourth sister—thank you. Because you and your documentary partners worked over time collecting, editing, and fine-tuning information about my life for a documentary about aging agelessly, you had a unique perspective like no other reviewer of my manuscript. Your comments led to a few strategically placed tweaks, resulting in clearing the path to allow readers to more easily supplant my experiences with internal strength life experiences of their own. As a result, hopefully readers will readily see themselves as having the type of powerful internal strength that it will take to establish and maintain a healthier lifestyle.

To Laurel Flax—thank you. You liberated my software at a time when all was almost lost. You saved pages and pages of text.

To each prevention-oriented health care team member— thank you. Time after time you supported my quest to prove that my nature-driven lifestyle defies medical science's research outcomes on aging and strength, flexibility, balance and energy.

To Patricia Ameling, eagle eye with an aerial view, thank you for your phenomenal feedback.

Epigraphs on Nature

In Lieu of a Preface

"Living in Nature, not with Nature is where the power lies."
—Richard Louv

"Come forth into the light of things, Let Nature be your teacher."
—William Wordsworth

"Earth and sky, woods and fields, lakes and rivers, the mountain and the sea, are excellent school masters, and teach some of us more than we can ever learn from books."
—John Lubbock

"Look deep into nature, and then you will understand everything better."
—Albert Einstein

"Nature holds all the answers—go outside and ask some questions—open your heart and listen to the response!"
—Amethyst Wyldyew

"I believe that there is a subtle magnetism in Nature, which, if we subconsciously yield to it, will direct us aright."
—Henry David Thoreau

"Never does nature say one thing and wisdom another."

—Juvenal

"The sun, with all those planets revolving around it and dependent on it, can still ripen a bunch of grapes as if it had nothing else in the universe to do."

—Galileo Galilei

"Nature is my medicine."

—Sara Moss-Wolfe

"If one way be better than another, that you may be sure is Nature's way."

—Aristotle

"Let us a little permit nature to take her own ways; she better understands her own affairs than we."

—Montaigne

"It's bizarre that the produce manager is more important to my children's health than the pediatrician."

—Meryl Streep

"Those who think they have no time for exercise will sooner or later have to find time for illness."

—Edward Stanley

"Take care of your body. It's the only place you have to live."

—Jim Rohn

"The future will belong to the nature-smart—those individuals, families, businesses, and political leaders who develop a deeper understanding of the transformative power of the natural world and who balance the virtual with the real. The more high-tech we become, the more nature we need."

—Richard Louv

Foreword

Those who are inspired by a model other than Nature, a mistress above all masters, are laboring in vain.

—Leonardo da Vinci

Leonardo da Vinci spent months studying birds in his attempts to understand how they fly. Even though he was unsuccessful in constructing a human flying machine based on nature's model of flying birds, da Vinci continued to admire nature's wisdom.

As early as the 1500s, da Vinci was practicing a process called biomimicry, a term which was not coined until the 1950s by American biophysicist Otto Schmitt. The word biomimicry comes from the Greek words "bios," meaning life, and "mimesis," meaning to imitate. Simply, I define biomimicry as human copying of nature's time-tested wisdom to make life much better by making it simpler and more sustainable for both humans and the environment. Inventors over many years have copied nature's wisdom in attempts to make life better for us all. For example, we all have used Velcro fasteners. Velcro was invented by Swiss engineer George de Mestral in 1941. Mestral got the idea directly from nature. His dog's fur was constantly stuck with burrs after romping outside. Mestral got tired of removing the annoying burrs from his dog's fur. Naturally curious, Mestral checked out the burrs through the lens of his microscope to see what was so unique about them and why they stuck to his dog's fur. He noted the tiny hooks on the end of the burrs' spines, which caught anything with a loop. That is why they caught his dog's fur and would not let go. From that knowledge and after years of experimentation, Mestral devised the opposite strips of a loose-looped weave that doggedly holds the hooks and earned US Patent 2,717,437. The saying "Necessity is the mother of invention" applies to Mestral's Velcro invention. (Bellis Updated 2016). The world beat a path to his door because his Velcro invention revolutionized the fastener industry.

After so many failed diets, my wondering ways eventually led me to check out nature's wisdom through my version of Mestral's microscope. Like Mestral and many other nature-based inventors, I found that nature's system-based, cycle-based, orderly, resilient, constant, responsive, simple, life-supporting wisdom could repair my out-of-control nutrition and movement lifestyle. The end result of my effort was uncovering Nature's Lifestyle Change System and its six-step formula. Applying the formula to my own life over time was just as innovative, sustainable, and achievable as Velcro. Since hope is what Nature's Lifestyle Change System and the six-step formula provides, I like Jonathan Sacks' quote on the mother of invention better. He said, "Hope, even more than necessity, is the mother of invention."

Précis

If you turned to this page, you are most likely thinking it wise to give Nature's Lifestyle Change System, with its six-step formula, a chance at repairing your lifestyle. After all, who can go wrong with nature's wisdom guiding the steps to a permanently healthier lifestyle? Nature programmed into the core of each step the capacity to assist followers to gain strength, flexibility, balance, and relaxation. The six all-inclusive steps take you from tapping into your internal strength at step one and relying on that strength to wade through the shoulder-high flood waters of step two, mind-body harmony. Steps one and two prepare you to tackle with passionverance the active requirements of step three, nutrition and movement. A genuine change in your nutrition and movement lifestyles prime you to step across the lifestyle change line at step four. By the time you reach step five, ongoing challenges, you will be equipped to turn setbacks into comebacks as you tackle nature's more intensive nutrition and movement challenges. New challenges will help you remain motivated. Step five is designed to prevent you from resting on your laurels, especially as you age. And finally, at step six you will enjoy overall healthier outcomes for the rest of your life.

Nature's Lifestyle Change System previously existed in an embryonic state. It was patiently waiting centuries for someone like me, capable of tuning into nature's wisdom intensely enough, to respect the astuteness of the system and to shake the six steps awake—and to do so at a time when they are needed most by society. The time is ripe, because according to the Centers for Disease Control and Prevention, a massive health tsunami is already upon us. Two-thirds of adults and one-third of children in the United States are in health trouble, simply because of their troubling lifestyles. In addition, the World Health Organization says that 40 percent of the world's population is overweight or obese. These disheartening statistics are powered by lifestyle choices.

Let us begin by looking at the significance of breaking away from the unhealthy herd to roam forever healthy in nature's lifestyle change herd. A lifestyle change under nature's wisdom means changes in the two most important lifestyle areas: nutrition and movement. Within nature's six-step formula are aids to provide you the support you need to make these changes. Running with the unhealthy herd will help you become a yo-yo diet expert. As you know, yo-yoing ignores the body's nutrition and movement needs in favor of taking the weight off no matter how. Yo-yoing usually results in not only temporary weight loss but unhealthy weight loss as well because critical muscle weight is lost rather than unhealthy fat.

Science agrees that the body is made up of eleven systems: nervous, skeletal, integumentary, muscular, endocrine, circulatory, respiratory, urinary, immune, digestive, and reproductive. Nature lets all who will heed her wisdom know that each of the body's systems is equally important; each system has been designed to work with all other systems for efficient functioning of the entire body.

Automobile systems, for example, are patterned after how the body was designed to function. We all know that if all auto parts are running efficiently, the car will run smoothly. If one part is not operating up to par, the car will not run smoothly, or not run at all, depending on which part is deficient. It is the same with the body. If the respiratory system, for example, is not up to par, the functioning of the entire body will not run smoothly, or not run at all, depending on the extent of the deficiency.

In laying out her plan to focus on nutrition and movement, nature pointed me to two qualities of success that she programmed into each of her creations. These two qualities are passion and perseverance. Passion and perseverance are nature's weapons of choice, as they work in tandem with her to meet her own challenges. They fit so snugly into nature's six-step formula that I coined the word "passionverance," symbolizing the fact that passion and perseverance are more powerful when applied together to meet life's challenges. Without both, challenges will go unmet.

Nature has already revealed the health realities with which you struggle because of your unhealthy lifestyle through her communications of pain and/or functional deficiency. Your doctor may also have uncovered nature's information about your health situation through examinations and lab tests. At any rate, you understand it is time for you to get serious about your health. So, this book does not preach to you about the importance of taking better care of yourself, especially now that you are older than you were yesterday. You already know the additional risks to health that aging brings. This book lays out how nature took hold and guided me all the way to super health. You can meet her requirements if you are willing to work hard to learn from my years of experiences. You will gradually follow nature's guidance all the way to a healthier lifestyle.

It took me years to break from the unhealthy herd with its false diet promises. Once free, I figured out and applied nature's powerful passionverance secrets. The developmental work and the informal trials are complete. The results are all in. After thirty years of living according to nature's six-step formula, I have become younger from the inside out at the cellular level, which is the most critical way to change a lifestyle according to the late Dr. Henry S. Lodge, coauthor of *Younger Next Year.* Lodge declares, "Most aging is just the dry rot we program into our cells by sedentary living, junk food, and stress." (Lodge 2007).

My results are verified by official medical exams, such as a healthy, strong resting heart rate that hovers around twenty-eight beats per minute, blood pressure readings hovering around 105/68, and X rays of my femur bones showing thickness rather than thinning, when I was in my sixties. In addition, blood panels taken before and after a six-day ultra-marathon foot race I ran in my early seventies showed thickening of my oxygen-carrying red blood cells in response to my muscles need for additional oxygen.

These are but a few of the healthy results because of my long-term lifestyle changes.

Know that your results will depend on the amount of time you devote and your beginning health and fitness levels along with the intensity of your passionverance levels. At a minimum, however, you could move closer to becoming healthier than you are at this moment. Anyone fortunate enough to understand and submit to the powerful benefits that nature provides (as I have) will automatically have access to a lifelong lifestyle that is healthy and fit despite aging.

If you choose to follow my example, you can begin to take full advantage of nature's wisdom as quickly as you wish. You won't need thirty years to figure things out. All you need do is to pack up your existing lifestyle, leave it outside, and move inside nature, where you can take the first step now.

Before the wheel was invented, people had no clue to what extent their lives would change for the better. It is the same with nature's six-step formula. The wheel's inventor came up against the same challenge that nature's six-step formula is now facing. Although nature's six-step formula was not invented by human hands, as the wheel was, both needed to explain the worth of something that never existed in society. Someone obviously did a praiseworthy job explaining the worth of the wheel, since it has affected civilization to the highest degree. In this book, I attempt to do an equally praiseworthy job of explaining the worth of nature's six-step formula to the health and well-being of society.

It is your decision. You can return this book to its place on the shelf alongside the type of books that led to your frustrations as you continue to struggle with your health, or you can buy this book and take a chance on nature's wisdom to help you establish and maintain *true* steps to a healthier lifestyle.

Contents

Part 3. *Nature's Six-Step Formula*

Introduction

In his book *Nature's Ways: How Nature Takes Care of Its Own*, Roy Chapman Andrews highlights how nature equips every creature with the capacity to obtain the necessities of life. Andrews believes that equipping creatures, even humans, with the necessities of life is nature's most fascinating aspect. (Andrews 1951). I found the aspect of nature taking care of its own to be fascinating as well. It is even more fascinating to me that so many people today simply ignore nature's offerings of nutrition and fitness, which are necessities of life. People are more in favor of speed and convenience to accommodate today's fast-paced lifestyles instead of taking advantage of nature's gifts of nutrition and fitness.

In times past, people seemed satisfied and healthier when indulging in nature's raw nutrition and labor-intensive ways of work, which kept them filled with energy throughout the entire day, from sunup to sundown. Raw nutrition meant that meals were composed of gathered fruits, vegetables, whole grains, legumes, seeds, nuts, and occasional animal protein, depending on the luck of hunters. In addition to ingesting nutrients to sustain life, grazing rather than eating three meals a day was the ideal way of eating. Moving most of the day and eating closer to nature's prepared foods was how early humans remained thin and relatively stress- and disease-free. For decades now, modern times have negatively influenced the human lifestyle. Today medical science attributes modern lifestyles for the massive increase in diseases or conditions such as certain cancers, heart disease, and type two diabetes.

I have very gradually taken nature up on her offer of the necessities of life and followed her lead for fitness, nutrition, and health, with tremendous results. The more I trusted nature, the more I worked with her directly, allowing her to become a living force in my life. This book is about my move back to nature's "raw" basics, and about how you can apply what I leaned to improve your health, despite the pull of today's modern world. In addition, you will not have to figure it all out over time as I did. The work has been done and nature's six-step formula awaits your participation.

Albert Einstein's genius is best known for influencing the methodology of all of science. Yet, he said, "I have no special talents. I am only passionately curious." Like Einstein, I am likewise passionately curious. But unlike Einstein, who not only had unquestionable credentials in his areas of expertise but was highly intelligent as well. I have no such conventional credentials in the nutrition or health professional fields. Woodrow Wilson best explained my IQ situation when he said, "I not only use all the brains that I have but all that I can borrow."

The United States Geological Survey (USGS), was created by an act of Congress in 1879. It has evolved over nearly 140 years and is the sole science agency for the Department of the Interior. USGS explained how deeply I became indebted to nature because I borrowed just about all that she had to lend. USGS points out that it is possible to:

Meet the world on its own terms, through a direct sensory experience. When this type of encounter is repeated over and over, day after day, deep connections form between the individual and place. Roots form on an emotional level as a sense of peace, curiosity, and wonder develop. At the same time, a network of new neural pathways in the brain is forming and the consciousness literally expands to encompass the rich variety of textures, scents, sounds, and images of nature. Lasting memories are formed during this type of deep sensory immersion. This is called primary learning—it takes place on a direct, visceral level.

Nature offers a rich complexity of ever-changing patterns. The textures and forms of the natural world appeal directly to the deepest aspects of human consciousness. At the most basic level, we are nature. There is no separation. We recognize that humans are part of the tapestry of life on this planet.

We recognize that our senses, minds, and bodies have developed in rhythm with the natural world; continual primary contact with nature is beneficial and needed for optimal health and well-being. Many studies demonstrate that obesity, depression, and other problems are linked with lack of time spent in the outdoors. This is called nature deficit disorder.

We have seen over 25 years the very positive results of providing youth and adults with regular, deep immersion experiences in nature in a safe, community-oriented setting.

I confess. I borrowed all that I could from nature. Living inside nature was like being on vacation where everything was new and fresh, beautiful and stunning, full of life and wonder, full of excitement but calming. What's more, living inside nature became my most comfortable way of life. Nature simply earned my trust. Unlike blindly following the unhealthy herd, with its "follow the leader" mentality, I was unrestricted in nature's vastness, her consistency, her creativity. I truly respected how nature operated. I soaked up all that nature taught me mostly through direct sensory experiences, without question or judgment.

Student of nature that I am, I continued learning about nature's wisdom as a member of the biology club in high school. The biology club probed deeper into the basis of nature's wisdom. Take nature's use of repetition as a teaching tool for example. We know from life's experiences that repetition is one of the simplest ways to learn something new. Repetition creates patterns which grabs attention. I believe that is why nature used repetition to help us simplify our complicated world.

For example, nature used repetition to teach about her use of geometric shapes. Some of nature's geometric shapes include waves and lines, pentagons, hexagons and spirals. Nature used the same handful of shapes over and over which created a pattern. It seems logical that nature's use of repetition gave birth to the field of biomimicry since inventors could easily explore the seemingly unlimited uses by nature of her geometric shapes.

Like all other shapes in nature, spirals, for example, exist everywhere. You can see them in weather patterns, sunflowers, the path of draining water, plant stems, snail shells, algae and ferns, to name a few locations. My biology club realized that spirals unleashed information about not only the beauty of such examples, but their many powers. Without repetition, I most likely would not have learned as much about the qualities of spirals.

It is a known fact in teaching fields that repetition can lead to understanding, can create familiarity, can get things into the long-term memory and it might even convince you to put all your eggs into nature's six-step formula basket. And remember that Paviov discovered how repetition can even connect a cue or trigger with a selected action.

My use of repetition throughout these pages hopefully will grab your attention as it helps bring the point home that the nature-based formula is not only new but is also superior to other health plans. But unlike most other plans, it is a lifestyle change program, not a diet. That it will take a combination of passion and perseverance (passionverance). That each step of the six-step formula is a stepping stone for the step after. That it is not easy to change a lifestyle, but hard work is the key. That nature is wise and building your lifestyle changes on her wisdom is worth a try. You will see that these concepts are repeated over and over throughout the book.

Part 1

Nature's Résumé

Man often becomes what he believes himself to be. If I keep on saying to myself that I cannot do a certain thing, it is possible that I may end by really becoming incapable of doing it. On the contrary, if I have the belief that I can do it, I shall surely acquire the capacity to do it even if I may not have it at the beginning.

—Mahatma Gandhi

Nature's Secret Ingredient

The greatest secrets are always hidden in the most unlikely places.

-Ronald Dahl

"Hey, Mom, you can't catch me," my daughter said as she took off running. I was twenty-nine years old, and she was only three years old at the time. Even though she was a young kid, she was right. I could not even catch my out of shape, cigarette-smoking breath much less her. In 1967, a year after she was born, and I had completed breast feeding, I started on the newly available prescription birth control pills. Two years later, I had doubled my weight to over two hundred pounds. The massive gain was one of many side effects of months on prescription birth control pills. My weight had spiraled completely out of my control.

Over a span of ten years, beginning in the early 1970s, I tried diet after diet and even prescription diet pills. Nothing, absolutely nothing, worked permanently. In fact, I ended up weighing more than when I started the first diet! I finally began to understand and accept that diets and other quick fixes were worthless because I happened to hear a local board-certified doctor, Dr. Gabe Mirkin (Dr. G.), on a radio show. He said,

> Eating is only part of a healthy lifestyle. You must add nutritious eating and movement if you wish to

achieve a healthy lifestyle. As for diets, you cannot go to bed forever hungry or unfulfilled. If you can't keep the weight off with a diet, know that you don't fail at dieting; dieting fails you. You are a success when you lose weight on a diet but are unable to keep the weight off. Diets were designed to help you do just that: take it off and gain more back. This happens over and over. For those unfamiliar, it is called yo-yo dieting.

Back in the 1970s, Dr. G practiced medicine way beyond his time. He preached about lifestyle changes as the only healthy means for a healthy life. I can still hear his passionate message:

> The only way to be both successful and healthy is to change your lifestyle in two critical ways. First, look at the food you've been eating. It should be made up of fruits, vegetables, whole grains, dried beans, seeds, and nuts—cutting back on animal products. The second way is to look at your movement habits. Your habits must get you out walking (or any other weight-bearing exercise of your choice) at least three days a week, gradually getting and keeping the heart rate up twenty beats above its resting rate, and keep it there for thirty minutes without stopping.

I followed his advice explicitly. Gradually over the years, I was able to go way beyond the doctor's advice, keeping off about eighty pounds, stopping smoking, and becoming fit enough to regularly engage in programs of walking, practicing tai chi and karate, swimming, and running. In fact, I became not only a runner but a marathon and ultra-marathon runner well into my seventies.

The more I followed the doctor's advice, the more I *wanted* to follow his advice. What's more, I was feeling better and had more than enough energy to keep up with my daughter, who by that time was a teen.

Many times, friends and family members asked:

> How can you change your lifestyle overnight just like that? You have been at this new lifestyle thing for a while with no hint of letting up. How do you handle your cravings for your bags of potato chips, your Three Musketeer's candy bars, your pints of black walnut ice cream, and your homemade German chocolate cake? Remember you even used to down the entire cake. And rather than sitting and eating your salty snacks while watching show after show on TV each evening as you used to, you are out some evenings walking, and running on other evenings, working hard on practicing tai chi or karate—and don't forget about your early morning swimming lessons on Wednesdays. I just don't understand what is making you change your lifestyle. You've got to have a secret. Please tell me what it is.

My early childhood home environment contributed to my optimism about life, which opens doors to passion, which opens other doors to internalize nature's teachings on perseverance. I grew up in the forties and fifties with five siblings (three sisters and two brothers), in a rural area where nature ran free and raw with fruit and nut trees and vegetable gardens. The nearby virgin woods held lessons on everything from astronomy to zoology. Our world was alive with birds, bees, bugs, worms, stars, flowers, weeds, sunshine, rain, the moon, hail, snow, rocks, dirt, and so on. It was filled with just about everything a child would want or need to learn. We all soaked up nature's teachings like sponges, from sunup until sundown, every day that we could. Nature's bounty in my neighborhood and in my extended back yard was free and limitless.

The very best part of spending so much time in nature's classroom was that life was timeless and each day was unscripted, so hurrying or becoming bored were not issues. Looking back, I can clearly see that passionverance was all that I would need many years later to take charge of my unhealthy lifestyle. It led the way to that first all-important step to change my lifestyle. And after taking the first step of nature's six-step formula, the other five steps seemed destined to follow.

Dr. G deserves all credit for telling me exactly what to do to become healthier by changing my lifestyle. However, he did not instruct in detail on exactly how to do it. I figured out with nature how to meet all of life's challenges, including my lifestyle challenges. So, nature deserves the credit for instilling in my deepest self the passion for guiding me to take on lifestyle challenges and teaching me to seal success by applying passion and the art of perseverance. Passion and perseverance together have been my motivating force through the direst straits or setbacks, no matter the odds or difficulties. Nature's six-step formula helped me overcome all obstacles that have come my way. Or at a minimum, if I found myself in disastrous circumstances, such as in the mists of overwhelming temptations, I had the internal strength to begin anew until the challenge was met. If you don't give up trying, you never fail. It is comforting and rewarding knowing that I carry the wherewithal inside of myself to overcome challenges; my mind is the keeper of my internal strength to make success happen.

There are many concrete examples of how nature relies on passionverance in her creations. The one creation that comes to mind is the dandelion. I liken my passionverance lines of attack to the passionverance approach taken by dandelions. Dandelions have survived and even become stronger, despite man's years of ongoing obliteration attempts and even today's modern weed killers. Cement sidewalks and motor-driven devices have not defeated them. That is why I call the dandelion the golden standard of nature's plant world and my secret lifestyle change ingredient.

Nature's Golden Standard

Like a dandelion up through the pavement, I persist.

—Stacy Cooper-Truex

A wise person once said, "May your search through nature lead you to yourself." Because of my daily access to nature in her most raw state, my inborn love for active observation of nature's doings, and the reactions my body encountered from my active personal interactions with nature, nature led me directly to myself. It was clear to me that the inner workings of nature's qualities of success were the powerful harmony of her passion and her perseverance. Nature's passion is present in all that she takes on, and all her masterpieces are rounded out by her perseverance. Again, everything in nature is harmonious and powered by both passion and perseverance—or "passionverance." My newly coined word—*passionverance*—reflects that harmony.

Looking back years later on my time spent with nature, I realized that I took on many of nature's traits. As a kid, passionverance influenced my way of thinking and living. It seemed the thing to do since nature's passionverance was very evident to me. I could hold in my small hands nature's golden standard, which later in life became my secret lifestyle change ingredient.

Before leaving my unhealthy lifestyle outside nature's front door, I found that I needed to prepare myself to take full advantage of what nature's wisdom on living a healthier life would require and provide. Some thirty years ago, just as I discarded the many diets and other so-called quick and easy solutions that failed me repeatedly, I began to see that I needed a means to bring my respect to light for not only living inside nature but also embracing her necessities as a lifestyle. My previous diets and experiences left me completely faithless in the worth of man-made solutions to the health pandemic raging out of control. Undertaking preparatory measures was like placing a down payment to secure my space inside nature's wisdom, which would give me full rights to access all that nature had to offer.

Fortunately, I grew up in a place where my parents educated me on things I needed to do well in school and become a productive member of society. Nature naturally took on the task of giving me the foundation for later school learning, simply by presiding over my outside play. In addition, my parents and siblings supported my play as well. I saw, felt, smelled, tasted, and heard nature daily for all my years growing up. I gained respect for all of nature's fury to her tranquility. I relied on nature, my best friend. Later, when I found myself heading for health trouble, it was not unusual for me to instinctively look to nature for exactly what I needed to establish an eating and movement lifestyle pattern that established and sustained excellent health.

By the 1970s, at middle age, I began taking steps to pack up my unhealthy lifestyle, leaving it outside nature's door and moving myself inside. That is when the grueling struggles with nature began. Those early struggles were powered by the modern world with its quick but unhealthy, and at times unsafe, products, in addition to the multi-billion-dollar advertisement budgets that convinced people that the unhealthy is healthy and the unsafe is super safe.

According to the USGS, it was my young years inside of nature that prompted me to finally close my mind to the inadequacies of the "quick-fix" modern world. In addition, my mind was also closed to family and friends who had no clue about the worth of my struggle to change my lifestyle. Somehow, my mind continued to be open to nature's soundness. Each day during the struggle, I subconsciously searched for nature's wisdom in everything. I could not connect any of the convenience foods or non-movement activities to nature's wisdom. I needed the ground and the sky and every plant and animal, which were inundated with passionverance. That is when I realized that the only way to set myself up for success was by bonding with nature's passionverance. Only then could I begin to take baby steps toward a healthful lifestyle.

First, I did not realize what nature had in store for me. I only knew that I knew nothing about the underlying reasons for nature's wisdom. That was wise, according to Socrates, who recognized that knowing when you do not know something is true wisdom. It took hindsight thirty years later to show me that nature's ways were not only to provide opportunities for me to gain the necessities of life but also to provide opportunities for me to function as a conduit that influences, inspires and stimulates all who wish to fully follow her wisdom. A clear picture of how nature had been prepping me throughout my life to take on the job of conduit as well, was revealed. I learned to take on the crusade not only to show that diets and other so called quick lifestyle health solutions are worthless, but also to be able to honestly relate "been there, done that" experiences to all who were at the same point relative to their failing lifestyles as I was. I found that my experiences served to motivate and inspire those who had wasted time and energy running with the unhealthy herd down that same worthless quick-fix path, reaping the same worthless results.

In my view, the dandelion inspires and motivates. It seems to have received the most demanding application of nature's six-step formula. In other words, nature bestowed upon the dandelion her most concentrated dose of passionverance. It takes a fortune of passionverance to thrive out of a tiny crack in the sidewalk.

Of all the creations in nature's kingdom, the dandelion caught my attention the most because of its properties. I believe it was their tufts of fluffiness that won me over as a child. As I grew older, I was intrigued to see those yellow pedals peeking out from between the cracks of the sidewalk in the city. I began to look forward to observing their ruggedness and their ability to survive despite impossible circumstances. I developed deep respect and gradually took on dandelion ways, which came with the safety net belief that I could push the limits of any challenge and succeed. The dandelion lifestyle model became my secret weapon in the fight against an unhealthy lifestyle. This connection allowed me to experience the rugged ability to thrive and flower no matter where the wind happened to sow my seeds. The major lesson I learned was that we humans can be much more resilient and ingenious than we ever thought we could be.

It seems that because of the connection with dandelions, my view of myself was automatically modified. Dandelions seem completely at peace with their plot. I too became a person who valued my inner intangible self, more than those tangible, material, man-made things that many others identify with. I see my mental muscle as a sum of every one of my experiences, mistakes, strengths, areas in need of improvement, thoughts, emotions, and bad habits, which means that occurrences such as these and many others are a permanent part of me.

Because of my organic view, passionverance has a solid foundation upon which to live and thrive deep within my makeup. I am reassured that whatever challenges the blowing wind may send my way, I will handle the test with passionverance much as the dandelion would.

The Eighth Wonder of the Natural World

Nature does nothing uselessly.

—Aristotle

We all agree that nature's inventiveness is limitless. Scientist, teachers, transit drivers, physical therapists, landscapers, computer programmers, farmers, lawyers, caretakers, law enforcement staff, and all others—even little kids—are rendered speechless when trying to explain nature's wisdom. To help make up for the loss of words to explain nature's genius, in my view, the staff at the Cable News Network (CNN) pulled together a list of some of nature's most breathtaking creations. The list is reminiscent of the list of the seven human-made wonders of the ancient world. Nature distributed these natural masterpieces throughout the world so more people could enjoy their beauty.

"Joy in looking and comprehending is nature's most beautiful gift," said Albert Einstein. The editors at CNN took Einstein's message to heart. Akin to the list of the seven wonders of the ancient world, in 1997 CNN created a list of the seven wonders of the natural world. The CNN editors were so enthralled with the brilliance and the massive natural beauty created by nature that they formulated the list to celebrate nature's incredible genius. CNN editors probably concluded that if humans highlighted their most impressive creations of the ancient world, certainly such a list for the natural world would be in order. CNN included on their list the following unbelievably breathtaking natural creations: Paricutin Volcano in Mexico, the Grand Canyon in Arizona, Victoria Falls (or Mosi-oa-Tunya or the Smoke That Thunders) in Zambia, Aurora Borealis (Northern Lights) in Canada, the Harbor in Brazil, the Great Barrier Reef in Australia, and Mount Everest in Nepal. (https://en.wikipedia.org/wiki/Seven_Natural_Wonders_%28CNN%29).

Nature, the architect of nature's six-step formula, began prepping me to uncover its existence back in the early 1970s. It took until the 1990s for me to gradually live and prove the worth of all six steps. This was too late for nature's six-step formula to be considered for the CNN list. Like the other natural creations on CNN's list, however, nature's six-step formula can have an enormous impact, not because of its breathtaking beauty as the others on the list boast, but because it will foster a healthy breath-giving lifestyle. If it is embraced by the human world, it will show nature at its most powerful and majestic, because it certainly has the potential of wiping out the lifestyle-driven health pandemic that is running rampant in the USA and beyond.

If the impact on my health and life is any indication of outcomes for all, it can make life healthier for the entire world. My results, which are defying medical science books on health and aging, are verified by my medical records. For example, my resting heart rate hovers around fit and healthy twenty-eight to thirty beats per minute. My red blood cells thicken to provide my working muscles more oxygen as I run ultra-marathons. My good cholesterol is nearly eighty. On X-ray, my femur bones have thickened as I age rather than becoming thinner. My blood pressure is well below the 120/80 mark. In addition, as a research study participant on aging and energy conducted by a widely respected research university, my energy levels rival fit people roughly thirty years younger. Because of my high level of fitness and health, I have had no flu, colds, aches, pains, or medications for over twenty-five years.

Some people, including some of my healthcare professionals, call me lucky to have such genes that allow me to go so far beyond what the medical books say about certain conditions and aging. But nature and I both know the reason for my good health, especially as I age. It is nature's passionverance at play which changed my lifestyle beginning thirty years ago.

While the seven natural wonders of the world play out on land, sea, or sky, the eighth wonder plays out inside the body of individuals wise enough to take the steps of nature's six-step formula. As such, the eighth wonder is foolproof and fail-proof, just like the dandelion.

Image of Nature's Wisdom

A picture is a fact.

—Ludwig Wittgenstein

It took decades working inside nature to create nature's six-step formula. My reward after so many years was that I was able to arrange nature's wisdom into a simple systematic process. Anyone with passionverance for lifestyle change can grab the opportunity for life-changing, better health. It is not easy to change a lifestyle in total; however, with nature's wisdom, it can be done. I did it!

The following paper reprinted with permission was written by Dr. Gabe Mirkin on why eat for health as you age. Dr. Mirkin lectured on this important topic on his radio show several decades before the research was reported in medical journals. I began to explicitly follow his advice on eating for health beginning in the early seventies. Today I continue eating only organic fruits, vegetables, whole grains, beans, seeds and nuts with astonishing health results.

Some pictures say more than a thousand words.

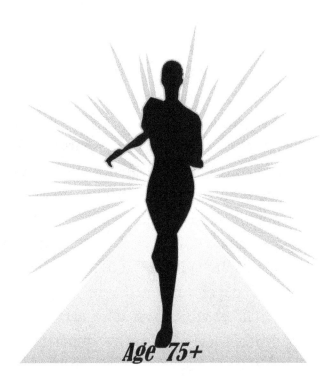

Age 75+

Healthy Aging and Senescent Cells
By Gabe Mirkin, M.D.
October 14, 2018

Extensive evidence shows that aging is associated with, and partially caused by, the accumulation of "senescent cells" in your body (*Curr Opin Clin Nutr Metab Care*, 2014;17:324–328). Recent animal studies have shown that it is possible to extend the lives of animals by reducing the numbers of senescent cells, even if treatment is started late in life (*Nature Medicine*, July 9, 2018).

What are Senescent Cells?

As you age, the cells in your body also age and many cells become "senescent cells". Normal cells go through a certain number of doublings and then are programmed to die. This is called apoptosis and is normal for all healthy cells. For example, the cells in your lips live only up to 48 hours, skin cells live up to 28 days, and red blood cells up to 120 days. As cells age, their DNA can be damaged so that they do not die (*Nestle Nutr Inst Workshop Ser*, 2015; 83:11–18). Senescent cells are not normal because they:

- try to live forever instead of dying at their programmed time
- stop producing new cells, and
- lose their ability to perform their normal functions.

For example, nerve cells lose their ability to transmit messages so you can become forgetful, uncoordinated, not able to move, or lose hearing or vision.

Most senescent cells are destroyed by your immune system in the same way it destroys bacteria and viruses. Your immunity recognizes bacteria and viruses that try to get into your cells by their surface proteins that are different from your normal cells. So your immunity makes white blood cells and chemicals called cytokines that attack and try to kill invading germs. In the same way, your immunity recognizes that senescent cells are different from normal cells and works to attack and kill them. Exactly the same cells and chemicals produced by your immunity to kill germs also are produced to attack and kill the senescent cells.

Senescent cells that are not destroyed by your immune system can become cancers (*PLoS Biology*, 2008; 6 (12): e301). Cancers do not become harmful as long as they stay in one place and do not overgrow a vital organ. For example, a woman does not die from breast cancer when it is limited to the breast. However, breast cancer cells can spread to the brain, bones, liver and other places to destroy these essential tissues and kill you.

How Do Senescent Cells Shorten Lives?

As you age, senescent cells start to accumulate in your body. This increase in senescent cells causes your immunity to stay overactive all the time in an effort to rid your body of the senescent cells. An immunity that stays active all the time is called inflammation, and your overactive immunity attacks not only the senescent cells, but also normal cells in your body. This damages healthy cells, so more and more cells become damaged and senescent, which is the very definition of aging (*Science*, 2006; 311: 1257). An overactive immunity can punch holes in the inner linings of your arteries, causing plaques to form which can then break off to cause heart attacks. An overactive immunity can also attack and damage the DNA in your cells to form even more senescent cells, which can overwhelm your immune system and increase the chances that these damaged cells will become established cancers.

Inflammation of aging is a primary driver for age-related diseases such as Alzheimer's disease and atherosclerosis (*Curr Pharm Des*, 2010;16(6):584-96). People who live to be 100 appear to be able to live longer than other people because they suffer less damage from their overactive immunities called inflammation (*Mech Ageing Dev*, Jan 2007;128(1):83-91). Centenarians may be at reduced and delayed risk for cancer because they have reduced markers of inflammation such as IGF-1 and p53 (*Cancer Immunol Immunother*, Dec 2009;58(12):1909-17).

Fruits and Vegetables to the Rescue

One effective way to reduce inflammation is to follow an anti-inflammatory diet. A diet that is loaded with fruits, vegetables and seeds and is low in added sugar, sodium and processed meats delays the markers of aging (*American Journal of Epidemiology*, October 1, 2018;187(10):2192–2201). As you grow older, the telomeres in cells shorten. Telomeres cover the tips of chromosomes in your cells and with each cell doubling, telomeres shorten, so doctors can measure aging by measuring the length of chromosomes in your cells. This study and others show that people who eat a high-plant, low-meat diet such as the DASH diet or Mediterranean diets have much longer telomeres than those who eat less healthful diets.

People who eat the most and widest variety of vegetables live the longest and have the lowest rates of heart attacks and heart disease (*Nutrition Journal*, July 10, 2018;17:67), most likely because fruits, vegetables and seeds are full of polyphenols and fiber. Polyphenols in fruits and vegetables reduced the number of senescent cells in mice to reduce disease and extend their lives (*EBioMedicine*, September

29, 2018). Furthermore, fruits, vegetables and seeds (beans, whole grains, nuts and so forth) have lots of soluble fiber, and bacteria in your colon ferment soluble fiber into short chain fatty acids that reduce inflammation and lower high blood pressure and cholesterol.

Dr. Mirkin's Recommendations

A major component of aging is the accumulation of senescent cells that stop performing their jobs that are necessary to keep you healthy. These cells then turn on your immunity to cause inflammation that can attack and destroy even more cells throughout your body. You can help to delay aging, prevent disease and live longer by following an anti-inflammatory lifestyle of:

- eating lots of fruits, vegetables, nuts, beans, whole grains and other seeds
- restricting red meat and processed meats, sugar-added foods, fried foods, and all drinks with sugar in them including fruit juices
- exercising
- avoiding overweight, particularly excess fat in your belly
- avoiding anything that damages cells such a smoking, drinking alcohol or exposure to other harmful chemicals

Reprinted with permission from Dr. Gabe Mirkin, Dr. Gabe Mirkin's Fitness and Health e-Zine

Part 2

Nature's Aids

Nature's Key to Wellness

Passion. It lies in all of us. Sleeping…waiting… and though unwanted, unbidden, it will stir…open its jaws and howl. It speaks to us…guides us. Passion rules us all. And we obey. What other choice do we have? Passion is the source of our finest moments…

—Joss Whedon

Perseverance is the ability to keep going in the face of continuous challenges. It is the ability to disregard distractions and to stay focused.

—Catherine Pulsifer

Nature's concrete version of passion and perseverance is the dandelion weed. Dandelions have much to teach us about benefitting from the use of passion and perseverance or, as I call it, *passionverance.* According to nature, using passionverance is the indisputable way to master every survival skill.

—B.H. Smith

Keith Wynn reminds us all that "Sometimes Mother Nature has the answers when you do not even know the questions". And Einstein adds, "We still do not know one thousandth of one percent of what nature has revealed to us". I agree one thousandth percent with both statements.

Back when I was a 200+ pound junk food eating smoker, I failed to turn to nature for answers to my out of control lifestyle. At the time, I simply did not realize that since birth, nature had provided humans all that they needed to live a healthy lifestyle—only if humans respected and followed nature's wisdom. Instead, like most others in my situation back then, I turned to the diet herd for help. After ten years of running with the diet herd, I ended up in worse health shape than when I started following the diet herd.

Because of my disappointment (read disgust) with the diet herd, I settled down and formulated one simple question. My question was, how do I establish and maintain a healthy lifestyle? With the help of the forward-thinking Dr. Gabe Mirkin who put me on nature's path to a healthy lifestyle, I began to look deeper and deeper into nature for answers to my health predicament and found nature's key, passionverance.

We all realize how difficult lifestyle habits are to break. There's always new lifestyle change challenges to attack. Food and fitness companies have the upper hand because they have spent and continue to spend trillions of dollars to convince you that your unhealthy lifestyle is not only convenient and can save you time but is also safe and healthy. Passionverance saved the dandelion weed from extinction. It can also save you from lifestyle-driven extinction if you are willing to take nature's six-step formula to heart. Nature programmed a potent dose of passionverance into each step of her six-step formula. Your job is to simply trust that nature has the answers to your health issues even if you do not know what questions to ask.

Nature's Wisdom and You

Introducing You to Nature's Lifestyle Change System's Six-Step Formula

> **Knowledge is having information. Intelligence is being able to use it to your advantage. Wisdom is being yourself in the process.**
>
> **--Unknown Author**

"Knowledge is having information"

The next section, Part 3 of Nature's Six-Step Formula, provides all the information that you need to become knowledgeable about taking pristine care of your health.

"Intelligence is being able to use it to your advantage"

As you work through each step of the Formula in Part 3, the process causes you to intellectually and totally activate the information to your advantage.

"Wisdom is being yourself in the process"

The examples given of my wisdom-filled life experiences set the stage for you to identify and wisely use your own wisdom-filled life experiences to be yourself in this lifestyle change process.

We all agree that nature is knowledgeable, intelligent and wise about all things. But most people may not realize (myself included years ago) how knowledgeable, intelligent and wise nature is about providing supports to help change lifestyles. Take nutrition, for example. I simply ignored all that I had learned from nature during my growing up years in favor of the diet herd with its man-made ingredients such as high fructose corn syrup that made apple pie and other diet herd "foods" tasty, speedy and convenient, but unhealthy. I failed to practice being myself—such as eating an apple directly from the tree. I ran with the herd for 10 long years before I traded in my diet disappointments and moved back inside nature's nutrition ways.

But all was not lost running with the diet herd. The major lesson that I learned running with the diet herd was that nature had all solutions to my health and fitness questions even when I did not know what questions to ask.

After I left the diet herd, I was open and free to easily access nature's ways in the many aspects of my life. In spite of all that nature has created since the beginning of time, she made it easy for me to access her gifts whenever needed. Ralph Waldo Emerson was a true fan of nature. He observed that nature's creations are easily accessed because they are organized according to natural laws and not according to luck.

In his book, <u>*The Laws of Spirit, A Tale of Transformation*</u>, Dan Millman discusses what I believe are twelve of nature's most important lifestyle change laws—balance, choices, process, presence, compassion, faith, expectation, integrity, action, cycles, surrender and unity. It seems that the underlying principle that ties these laws together is movement. It is as if nature did not allow her creations to become stagnant.

Each law is important, and all must be followed to live the most vibrant, well-balanced, healthy life possible. The laws of cycles helped me see how unwise following the diet herd was with its unsystematic, static tactics. I did not realize it at the time, but looking back on my life, I could clearly see that because of my overwhelming frustration with the diet herd, I was searching for a no-nonsense way to a healthier life. That is when I began following nature's lifestyle change laws, focusing on laws of cycles which focused on her systems of gradual progress and her one breath, one step at a time best practice. Amazingly, my healthier lifestyle began to gradually unfold in step with nature's six-step formula. Millman succinctly captures the central points of laws of cycles in the introduction to his chapter on Cycles:

> "The world of nature moves in rhythms, patterns, and cycles—the passing of the seasons, the movement of the stars, the ebb and flow of the tides. The seasons do not push one another, neither do clouds race the wind across the sky. All things happen in their own

good time—rising and falling and rising like ocean waves, in the circles of time."

Nature's water cycle which is driven by the heat energy of the sun, is one of nature's more complicated cycles to observe. Water changes states among liquid, gas and ice at different places in the cycle—evaporation, condensation, precipitation, run-off and ground water. It is quite interesting to note that there has been the same amount of water on earth for millions and millions of years because the total amount of water on earth remains constant. Prehistoric humans may have washed themselves in a stream that contained the same water that you now use to brush your teeth!

Nature's Lifestyle Change System's six-step formula mimics the butterfly's life cycle which is one of nature's most straight-forward cycles to understand and observe. Many of us observed the life cycle of the butterfly in middle or high school biology class. We readily followed the butterfly's journey through four separate stages in its life cycle. It begins life as an egg at stage one. By stage two, the egg hatches and becomes larva (caterpillar). By stage three, it relaxes inside a pupa (chrysalis) at complete rest. Finally, at stage four the colorful flying adult butterfly emerges from the pupa. The butterfly's life cycle is very controlled, very organized and very predictable.

Nature's Lifestyle Change System is likewise very controlled, very organized and very predictable. Like the butterfly's life cycle, each step of the six-step process is different and serves a different purpose. Also, like the butterfly's life cycle, each step of the six-step process serves as a conduit that helps power the next step in the lifestyle change process. While passionverance is an automatic part of the butterfly's makeup, nature tells us that humans must identify from deep inside of themselves and engage internal strength forceful enough to open doors to passionverance. Passionverance can in turn provide successful cycling through all six steps of Nature's Lifestyle Change System.

The stronger your internal strength, the wider the door to your passionverance will swing open. In other words, having strong internal strength forces the mind and body to work together in harmony, which intensifies passionverance, making it less taxing to achieve challenge after challenge. At this early point in your struggle, however, as I was so long ago, you may not have faith that the strength of your internal strength is strong enough to open passionverance's door. Under nature's guidance, I learned to access and strengthen my internal strength. It all started when I went back in time in my mind to the couple of times in my life when my internal strength flexed its strongest muscles. Such strength automatically turned on my passionverance. The first time was when I helped to integrate the local high school. And the second was when I was too unhealthy to play a simple game of tag with my three-year-old. I finally realized that I was in my own way both times and could not take full advantage of all that life had in store for me. To move myself out of my own way, I needed to make drastic changes in my approach to life. Such far-reaching changes, I knew, would call for digging down deep inside to grab ahold of the strongest internal strength I could reach. Once there, I held on tightly to that strength and was able to unlock passionverance's door which in turn housed the grit I needed to move myself out of my own way. In a mostly hostile school environment, I changed my entire approach to integrating the country's number one ranked public high school. As a result, I achieved more of what that school had to offer. And seven years later, I took the first baby step towards changing my whole lifestyle to become a positive force in my daughter's life as a fit and healthy new mom. As a result, not only did my strong internal strength open the doors to my strongest passionverance, it gave me the power to work hard to overcome both challenges. My passionverance continued to strengthen through every challenge since.

Trust that deep passion for change automatically produces the internal strength that you will need to power your passionverance before you can begin to conquer challenges. That is to say, if you are deeply passionate about taking better care of yourself as you cycle through each step of the process, your internal strength will continue to rise to the level that is needed to meet each lifestyle change challenge. Again, nature made it such that the deeper your level of passion about lifestyle change, the stronger your passionverance. All you must do is keep your focus true to the task. Remember, initially you may not have faith that the strength of your internal strength is strong enough. Your passionverance will strengthen as you work through each step in the process.

An English proverb reminds us that the caterpillar thought the world was over when it became a butterfly. To keep you solidly on target as you cycle through, allow the butterfly to remind you not to give up too soon and to adopt the pace of nature: her secret is patience. Your patience will carry you through each step of nature's six-step formula beginning with step one.

Step One of Nature's Lifestyle Change System

Step one of Nature's Lifestyle Change System's six-step formula, internal strength, houses the source of your success in accomplishing the challenges imbedded in each step of the process. Identifying and relying on your internal strength is where you will become yourself in the process because you will grab and hold fast to the passion involved in one (or more) of your most difficult past challenges. Your internal strength was so strong during your past struggle that you overcame the challenge against all odds. It was your genuine moment of truth.

Think back to that time in your past when your internal strength flexed its strongest muscles. That was most likely a time when you wanted to change something so badly that you could almost taste the change. Go back to that time in your mind, feel the passion you felt then and hold fast to that passion. That passion will be your one-way ticket to board the train heading for lifestyle change today. It was a challenge that caused you to gather, from deep inside of yourself, every last ounce of your internal

46

strength which called up passionverance. We all have at least one such challenge that we mastered that told us exactly who we were and what we were made of. You could have directly or indirectly experienced the challenge, or maybe it was a health issue that you fought and survived after your doctors had given up all hope. This challenge could have dragged you below ground where the sun never shines, but you were able to claw your way back up to the sunshine. It most likely was so overpowering that it changed you and your life for the better. It stood out way beyond all of your many other challenges because you had to dig your deepest to achieve it. It could have become worthy of becoming your yard-stick against which you could forever say, "If I achieved that challenge, I know I can achieve all others". Hold fast to that passion and its accompanying passionverance as you cycle through steps two to steps six of the process.

Step Two of Nature's Lifestyle Change System

Your stronger internal strength will begin to push open the door to passionverance at this step. You will begin cycling through step two of Nature's Lifestyle Change System's six-step formula, mind/body harmony. Nature will not assume that you know the importance of your mind and body working together as close allies. That is why your first action under this step will be to understand that your mind and body are so connected that they are inseparable.

Passionverance's support is 100 times more robust when you work mind and body as a single unit. To keep you solidly on target as you cycle through the remainder of step two, allow the butterfly to remind you to never give up trying by adopting the pace of nature: her secret is patience.

Step Three of Nature's Lifestyle Change System

Steps one and two prepared you for step three, the "super bowl" of Nature's Lifestyle Change System's six-step formula, nutrition/movement harmony. Of all of the steps in the process, step three is your proving ground. Your time of truth, the point where you get down to brass tacks, the real heart of it all, where you become healthier than your very best excuse for falling off the wagon.

You will begin learning new information about the importance of nutrition and movement working in harmony as you cycle through. Studies show that understanding comes before acceptance and only genuine acceptance leads to genuine action. Therefore, your first lesson will be that nature will not assume that you know the importance of nutrition and movement working together as allies. From this point in the process, you will be advised to cease isolating one from the other. You will learn the underlying reasons why it is critical to tend to nutrition and movement challenges simultaneously.

Remember, most diet herd methods only deal with food, hardly ever food and movement.

Passionverance's support is 100 times more robust when you work nutrition and movement as a single unit. To keep you solidly on target as you cycle through the remainder of step three, allow the butterfly to remind you to never give up trying by adopting the pace of nature: her secret is patience.

Step Four of Nature's Lifestyle Change System

Your internal strength will be the strongest ever now that you will have completed three of the six steps in the process. You will begin cycling through step four of Nature's Lifestyle Change System's six-step formula, lifestyle change line. Now, most lifestyle change struggles cease. You will begin to relax and allow nature to take over providing you spontaneous support gifts you will automatically use not only to maintain your new healthier state, but to continue to improve it forever.

Here is a sample of the support gifts you can expect nature to provide. All of the calories you were not burning before will no longer be stored as fat. They will simply disappear because you will lose that excess weight. Your mind will make you feel good about losing weight which lessens craving for high fat junk foods. You will not tire as easily during your daily living activities. You may not realize it, but the inside of your body will make drastic health changes as well. Your medical tests will begin to show that your blood sugar and insulin levels have stabilized. Your blood pressure, cholesterol and resting heart rates will cease creeping upward. Your mental state will lift, and your self-concept will suffer less because you will be feeling so much better about yourself. Also, you will cease having low periods because nature's gifts will help change your pessimistic mind-set regarding control of your health. You will begin to see yourself as being solidly in control of your health.

You will also find that nature will let you know exactly how you are doing by communicating messages via your physical body. Either your physical body will feel no pain as you move along smoothly since it is working like a well-oiled machine, or it will begin to feel pain because one part or another is out of whack. Your job will be to continuously scan your body from top to bottom to determine how you are doing. If you stray, even temporarily from the program, nature will be right there whispering her discontent that you can physically feel through pain. The pain might be in the form of a sore muscle, indigestion or a belly ache depending on which body part is involved. For example, if you eat too much or eat the wrong foods, nature's message might be in the form of a belly ache followed by diarrhea, or you might just get that squeezy feeling inside that you get when you just don't feel like your normal self.

Nature has a way of communicating slight issues by whispering softly at first. Hopefully, you will take heed in response to nature's soft whisper. But if you do not, she will continue to intensify her whisper which means that the pain will in turn intensify. And if you continue to ignore nature's message that something is out of whack and you need to take quick action—she will begin to scream her loudest, making the pain so unbearable that a doctor's or hospital visit is your only option for relief.

Nature's wisdom will allow you to live peacefully according to your new ways of eating and moving as long as you stick with the program. But know that nature will not let you rest on your laurels for long. To keep you solidly on target as you continue to cycle through the remainder of step four, you will forever be forced to take on more aggressive food and movement challenges. Always allow the butterfly to remind you to never give up trying by adopting the pace of nature: her secret is patience.

Step Five of Nature's Lifestyle Change System

You will begin cycling through step five of Nature's Lifestyle Change System's six-step formula, ongoing challenges. Your internal strength will open the door to your deepest level of passionverance thus far. Passionverance will provide you the best possible support since it will have you forever searching for your next nutrition and movement challenges. Nature's wisdom will tell you that you must continuously up the ante by accepting newer and newer challenges. Upping the ante will help you remain inspired, motivated, determined, interested, excited and encouraged to continue the hard work that it will take to continue to reap healthier outcomes. To keep you solidly on target as you cycle through the remainder of step five, allow the butterfly to remind you to never give up trying by adopting the pace of nature: her secret is patience.

Step Six of Nature's Lifestyle Change System

You will forever and ever cycle through step six of Nature's Lifestyle Change System's six-step formula, healthier outcomes. Because you will have conquered all six steps—internal strength, mind/body harmony, nutrition/movement harmony, lifestyle change line, ongoing challenges and healthier outcomes—you will know that you have arrived since you will be solidly on the road to a healthier you. The six steps will forevermore band together in your sub-conscious mind to provide you a permanent lifestyle of strength, flexibility, balance and relaxation across nutrition and movement.

Every day, you will feel better, look better, have more energy and receive healthier reports from your health care team. Friends and others will notice the new you. Some will demand to know your secret. To keep you solidly on target as you live your new life, allow the butterfly to remain your best friend. Congratulations! Your new Lifestyle by Nature is the new you—forever.

Take the introductory information in this part with you to the next section, Part 3, Nature's Six-Step System. It will help set the stage for the hard work that will be required as you put into action steps one to six of the lifestyle change process. A friendly butterfly appears in the background on each page of the next section. It is there as a constant reminder to guide you through each step of your metamorphosis and to remind you to hold on to the pace of nature.

The Big Picture at a Glance

At a glance, the matrix below succinctly highlights the framework of Nature's Lifestyle Change System which includes the skill goals and function zones of each of the six steps. Continuously refer back to this matrix because it will keep you on track as you proceed through the requirements of each step in the process.

Framework of Nature's Lifestyle Change System

The Six-Step Formula's Skill
Goals and Functional Zones

The Six Step Formula	Step #1 Internal Strength	Step #2 Mind/Body Harmony	Step #3 Nutrition/ Movement Harmony	Step #4 Lifestyle Change Line	Step #5 Ongoing Challenges	Step #6 Healthier Outcomes
Skill Goals	To revisit a past time when you conquered your most difficult "against all odds" challenge.

To harness the powerful internal strength, it took to meet the "against all odds" challenge.

To call on your powerful internal strength to open the door to your powerful passionverance | To absorb nature's wisdom on mind/body harmony and incorporate its essence into your regular lifestyle change practices | To absorb nature's wisdom on nutrition and movement harmony and incorporate its essence into your regular lifestyle change practices | To absorb Nature's wisdom on lifestyle change support gifts and incorporate its essence into your regular lifestyle change practices | To absorb nature's wisdom on ongoing challenges and incorporate its essence into your regular lifestyle change practices | To congratulate yourself as you continue to roll up your sleeves to hold on to nature's wisdom and your new healthier lifestyle forever |
| Functional Zone #1 | Reflect on the strength of your internal strength and transfer that strength and power to your passionverance | Experience your most powerful passionverance which allows you to establish and maintain nature's wisdom on mind/body harmony | Experience your most powerful passionverance which allows you to establish and maintain nature's wisdom on nutrition/ movement harmony | Experience your most powerful passionverance which allows you to establish and maintain nature's wisdom on lifestyle change support gifts | Experience your most powerful passionverance which allows you to establish and maintain nature's wisdom on ongoing challenges | Experience your most powerful passionverance to live contently in your new lifestyle forever |

Lifestyle by Nature   Betty Holston Smith, Ed.D.

The Six-Step Formula's Skill
Goals and Functional Zones

The Six Step Formula	Step #1 Internal Strength	Step #2 Mind/Body Harmony	Step #3 Nutrition/ Movement Harmony	Step #4 Lifestyle Change Line	Step #5 Ongoing Challenges	Step #6 Healthier Outcomes
Functional Zone #2	Let your harnessed most powerful internal strength open the door to your most powerful passionverance	Move yourself inside nature's wisdom and trust her wisdom on the efficiency of mind and body functioning as one	Move yourself inside nature's wisdom and trust her wisdom on the efficiency of nutrition and movement functioning as one	Move yourself inside nature's wisdom and trust her wisdom on the efficiency of using nature's support gifts to forever remain on target	Move yourself inside nature's wisdom and trust her wisdom to lead the way to your acceptance with open arms of new and difficult challenges in your nutrition and movement lifestyle	Move yourself inside nature's wisdom and trust her wisdom to lead you to remain inspired, motivated, determined, interested, excited and encouraged to continue the hard work it will take to continue to reap healthier outcomes forever
Functional Zone #3	Allow the power of passionverance to continuously attack and conquer the lifestyle challenges inherent in the next step in the six-step process	Allow the power of passionverance to continuously attack and conquer the lifestyle challenges inherent in the next step in the six-step process	Allow the power of passionverance to continuously attack and conquer the lifestyle challenges inherent in the next step in the six-step process	Allow the power of passionverance to continuously attack and conquer the lifestyle challenges inherent in the next step in the six-step process	Allow the power of passionverance to continuously attack and conquer the lifestyle challenges inherent in the final step of the six-step process	Allow the power of passionverance to continuously attack and conquer the lifestyle challenges you will continuously meet as you age

Part 3

Nature's Six-Step Formula

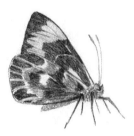

I have always loved butterflies, because they reminded us that it's never too late to transform ourselves.

—Drew Berrymore

Step One of Nature's Six-Step Formula: Internal Strength

Only in the midst of challenging moments do you find your inner strength.

—Author Unknown

Internal strength opens the door to passionverance. The stronger your internal strength, the wider the passionverance door will spring open. If passionverance is absent from any changes that you wish to make, you are fooling yourself; you simply won't be able to make the change permanently. Qualities such as willingness to take risks and thriving on pressure, optimism, empathy, resilience, and courage are the ingredients that make up internal strength. And your internal strength will give you the power to fight against your many years of bad lifestyle habits. Know that you have been cultivating your own internal strengths, usually by overcoming all types of life-altering challenges, throughout your life. Every challenge that you have overcome was because you used your internal strength to fight and win the battle.

I found my most robust inner strength in the mist of my most robust challenge, which ended to be my most life-altering experience. Most people have at least one challenge that they can point to that was life altering—the type of challenge that shows you exactly who you are and what you are made of. I had such an experience that revealed to me that I had the internal strength to survive against all odds. My internal strength was reminiscent of the internal strength given to the dandelion by nature.

When I was about fourteen years old, Daddy put his foot down and my whole world fell apart. I was forced by him to go to the local public high school. The new school had over three thousand students, and my existing school had only a few hundred students. Even today, I can still hear my father say, "School integration is a huge step forward for our race. Just think, Betty, you will go to the highest-ranked public high school in the entire country! Our lives are drastically changing, and it's a great time to be alive to experience this great change. You will be able to give your grandchildren eyeball accounts of how it all happened."

The year was 1956, and on that first day of school, my mother drove me to the senior high school in Maryland, just north of the Capitol of the free world. I remembered feeling secure in the front seat of my mother's car as I looked at the school for the very first time. I saw a huge, intimidating campus with buildings sitting well back from the street. It was nothing like my other school with its one building. A long sidewalk that led to stairs up to the entrance seemed miles and miles long. Off to the left, just below the first step, was a chalkboard with the word "Welcome" in bold letters. I remember that the word only momentarily settled my stomach; between me and the front door were seemingly thousands of kids, but my survey didn't pick out anyone in the crowd who looked anything like me. Silent tears streamed down my face. I remember turning to look at my mother a last time—a final quiet plea before leaving her car, to be returned to my smaller, secure, black school located ten miles north.

"Betty, your father and I know how scared you are, but we also know that you will tackle your fears and do just great because you are so strong," my mother said. For the millionth time, mother's upbeat encouragement didn't work.

Since 1776, discrimination had been skillfully executed by American society because framers of the Constitution of the United States of America saw my race as inferior. The laws governing school segregation had recently changed in 1954, but what would have made these students, or this faculty think or act any differently only two years later? We all know that laws can change, but it does not mean that people's hearts change. The root of my fear was embedded in what I called the "dichotomy of my life": seeing myself as first class in my own family as well as my black world, while struggling against the second-class label put upon me everywhere else.

With notebook in hand, I left my mother's car to begin what I believed was my unjust punishment because I was born a Black American. Suddenly, each foot turned into a one-ton cement block. Thunk, thunk—the sound each foot made as I dragged one foot then the other to the school's door. As I got closer, it became the only sound. I remember that the kids abruptly stopped greeting each other after the long summer break to stare at me. The wind stopped blowing. The sun hid behind a cloud. Even the birds stopped singing.

Thunk, thunk.

I remember thinking that I simply did not belong in this white school with other white kids. Black kids just did not go to school with white kids—it was simply unheard of. And at that time, I thought that I did not deserve to be going against the way things were since I was born. I could not picture myself the "inferior human" sitting next to them in the classroom or eating next to them in the cafeteria or, God forbid, showering with them in gym class.

I finally made it to the chalkboard. There was no welcome or any other message for me there. So, I continued up the steps and through the door.

Thunk, thunk.

Hundreds more kids were standing around inside, and when they saw me, there was the loudest silence I had ever heard.

I entered the office and stood there, hugging my notebook like it was my lifeline—and it was. The "thunk, thunk" stopped, and I noticed that the loud silence got even louder. Three white women stopped their conversation midsentence and stared at me from behind the counter. One asked my name, and another asked if I was lost. I somehow found my voice, although barely above a murmur. I gave my name and even managed to ask for directions to my homeroom. But deep down I was screaming, "Yes, I'm lost! I've been very lost in discrimination all my life. In addition, that is why I fear integrating this school, with its all-white faculty and the 3,500 white students." I felt way out of my "colored" place.

My fears, I soon discovered, were not in vain. I was openly and harshly mistreated by some of the kids and covertly by some of the teachers. I cried every evening at home for most of that first year. My grades went from A's and B's to mostly D's. I was miserable. You see, my attitude toward my involvement in this school was as pessimistic as my attitude was twelve years later toward being successful in taking and keeping eighty pounds off my weight. At the onset, they both were so hopeless that even a million dollars would not have altered my attitude one iota. The few steps down that sidewalk to that chalkboard and up those steps to that door were by far the most difficult things I had ever done up to that point. In fact, I still measure the difficulty of my life's challenges against being integrated into that school. I really learned so much about life and about myself during my struggles that first year and later when I began to have some positive experiences. I came out of it a much better person.

A smart person once said that growth can only begin when you start to accept your own weaknesses. I really don't know when I started observing my view of myself as looked at through the eyes of whites as my own weakness—but I did. Looking back, I figured out that it was the lessons learned from the dandelion that helped me to be at peace with my true ranking as a human being. Once I accepted responsibility for the misconstrued view that I held of myself, I began to change my attitude toward the entire experience. Only then was I able to grow at that school that had everything imaginable for high-quality learning.

I was part of the problem; I was in my own way. Among other things, I expected the school to take all responsibility for my plight. I thought that I should be able to sit back and let the school officials sort of "do unto me," rather than my taking the responsibility to "do unto myself." So from the very beginning, my expectations of the experience were colored by a very negative attitude. Whatever the reasons— society's segregation laws, youth, fear of the unknown, inexperience—I was put into a place that I could not see my way out of until the experiences of the change itself sort of took me by the shoulders and said, "Get a grip or you won't make it through."

By the beginning of my second year there, I "got a grip," which resulted in a huge turnaround in my attitude. I began to take responsibility for how I viewed my own worth as a person, a human being, a student, who up to that point was in a segregated but unequal school. Over time, I found out that the best learning is derived from the roughest parts of life's experiences. Believe me—I had clawed way up the rough side of that integration mountain.

With my changing attitude, I was able to take more productive advantage of most that the school had to offer, except when barriers were thrown in my way by the few diehard segregationist kids, teachers, or counselors. In fact, one counselor advised me to switch from the academic program to the commercial program. Her reasoning was that I did not have the brain power to succeed in college, and even if I did, my parents could not afford to send me to college. She thought it would be much better for me to learn to type, take shorthand and qualify for a clerical government job—the only office job available to a young Black clerical office worker in the 1960's. She wrongly thought that I aspired to become a typist because she thought that I was not smart enough to go beyond. Let me clarify, typing is a great job, especially forty years ago. However, the counselor did not know my parents or had no clue about the importance of education in my daily home life.

I learned the hard way that sometimes in life seemingly negative situations result in positive good. Those barriers the counselor and others put in my way were super negative. But I followed through as the counselor said: I switched to the commercial program, was graduated from that school on time, passed the federal civil service test as a typist, and was hired in my first typing job after high school for the United States government. The counselor had no clue that the job was so boring that I simply hated it.

On my first day at work, I knew that I was in the wrong job. The positive part was that I was motivated to enroll in evening classes in college after work. I completed my undergraduate degree, a master's degree in business and public administration, and a doctorate—all during part-time studies over a thirty-two-year span of time. An even more positive part was that the more solid those barriers, the harder I worked to go over, under, around, or smash my way through them. I grew stronger and stronger each time I met and surpassed those negative challenges to my learning.

I look back at those times through today's lens of Richard Louv's work on nature-deficit disorder. I believe that spending much of my pre-adult years outside in nature are part of the reason why I was calm enough to focus on standing up to the integration battles head on. I was free to focus the bulk of my energy on my safety and welfare. Louv, the author of the bestsellers *Last Child in the Woods* (2005) and *The Nature Principle* (2011), coined the term "nature-deficit disorder". In a talk at National Geographic Headquarters in Washington, D.C, Louv explained the term "nature-deficit disorder".

I simplified his explanation of deficit disorder as being stuck in a place where dirt has been buried under man-made cement, vegetation has been blocked out by black-out shades, or the sky has been traded for sky-high skyscrapers.

I believe that the force of my internal strength was revealed to me as alive and kicking during the last two of my high school years. Louv's research on the importance of nature's influence on living uncovered part of the reason for my strong internal strength at such a young age. I believe that because I grew up in a family living the core values demonstrated by mother and daddy, the foundation of my energetic internal strength became part of my DNA since I had the best of both nature and nurture worlds.

Because I was able to change my attitude regarding my dilemma, the dilemma itself changed—it went from negative to positive. When you find a way to look differently at something, that something changes. I encourage you to look differently at your current health, fitness, and nutrition circumstances, so your task to take better care can become manageable. Remember, I was able to make this change at a very young age. I believe that you will be able to change your attitude regarding the difficulty of taking better care of yourself as a more mature person.

The essence of what my integration experience symbolized was that I underwent a significant change in my mindset. And you must figure out for yourself what you must come to grips with to change your mind about permanent lifestyle changes. I'm sure that you have a life-altering experience that you can point to that provided you the same type of negative/positive experience you can use to hold on to as you change your mindset.

Later in my life, I understood what that dandelion's appeal was all about and why I was so connected to it. It was revealed to me that nature's six-step formula was going to be my saving grace. Internal strength saved me from the integration turbulence, just as the dandelion's internal strength saved it from obliteration.

I did not know that I needed to focus on internal strength or that it had anything to do with pointing the way to passionverance. In all of my readings, as I looked for real help, I never read a thing about the need to have strong internal strength to open the doors to passionverance, the driving forces behind lifestyle change. For this type of permanent change, the type that qualifies as real lifestyle change, you need to make sure that your machine has smooth-moving parts. Without internal strength to provide access to your passionverance, you simply will not go very far in nature's six-step formula.

Remember, you have been cultivating and relying on these qualities since you were conceived. You might not recall learning to sit up, scoot, crawl, balance, or walk. You most likely fell hundreds of times in the process. But you obviously also got up hundreds of times. After all, you learned to walk. Each time that you stood again, you strengthened your internal qualities. You called on them and strengthened them as a kid when you learned to ride a bike. If you fell off one hundred times, you got back on the bike at least 101 times. You strengthened them even more to finish high school and educate yourself beyond—to meet all your life's challenges no matter how difficult. Without passionverance you cannot really succeed at anything in life. You likely have not realized that each success depends on the strength of your internal strength—neither did I until I realized how hard I was willing to work to succeed whenever I had clear intentions to succeed. Until internal strength opens the door, you have no idea about how strong you are.

⚠ You must keep pushing harder today than you pushed yesterday to guarantee healthier tomorrows. It takes a wealth of butterfly-type patience and dandelion-type passionverance to successfully reap healthier lifestyle outcomes for the rest of your life. Remember. Using nature's principles of patience and passionverance will allow you to expertly internalize the important information presented in this section. Know that the information presented here becomes the core of the next step in the process. It is also important to note that at each step you are gradually required to be yourself in this process.

Part 3

Step Two of Nature's Six-Step Formula: Mind–Body Harmony

There is a lot of scientific evidence that shows the chatter between mind and body goes two ways.

—University of Chicago

Passionverance opens the doors to step two of nature's six-step formula: mind–body harmony. It is critical for your mind and body to work in harmony to become actively involved in your change hopes and dreams. It is key for you to know that your mind and body are actively involved and both depend on each other to affect permanent changes in your unhealthy lifestyle habits.

Most of us have experienced up close how nature provides her living creatures with the capacity to obtain the necessities of life. I believe that obtaining the necessities of life is so important that nature programmed into our minds and bodies the capacity for the mind to influence the body, and vice versa. In other words, the human mind and body are interconnected in a communication link. Mind and body linked together are very powerful. The power is evident in the effort they exert together to help you meet life's challenges. Sian Beilock, a former psychology professor at the University of Chicago, believes the mind–body connection starts early and continues to the end of life. (Beilock 2015, 6).

Experts believe your mind is where all changes must originate. If your mind is not molded to make change, permanent change can never take place. Through your thoughts and emotions, your mind speaks to you constantly. For example, as you cycle through the change process, you will find your thoughts and emotions work in harmony to keep you focused on the ultimate prize. Your mind might make you feel guilty because you ate something that you should not have, or you cut your exercise routine short without a good reason. Listen to your mind, take note, and then act. Your body acts on changes that your mind demands, and your mind acts on changes that your body demands.

Your mind and body can either support your goals and help to conquer challenges or not. Most people don't know the power that can be brought to bear to achieve all manner of challenges because most people aren't conscious of this mind-body power. They do not realize that they can have a better chance of meeting life's challenges and reducing stress in the process if the communication link is routinely called upon as part of daily living. To have the best of your health in tow, for example, you need to understand, accept, respect and act on the power of the mind–body communication connection and then build a harmonious relationship between the two.

Mind–body experts such as the late Kenneth Pelletier, MD, was a leader in the field of mind–body medicine and author of *The Best Alternative Medicine (Pelletier 2000) Sound Mind, Sound Body (Pelletier 1994)* informs us through his writing about the invisible communication link between the mind and the body and the body and the mind. Pelletier believed that this link is programmed into the human DNA at the time of conception. I believe that this communication link is like the instincts that nature programs into plants and animals. But an animal's or plant's instinct is automatically activated when needed, whereas the communication link in humans must be called upon challenge by challenge to become recognized. Turning the link on can change mindsets from negative to positive, which tells the body to behave in a positive rather than a negative manner. Simply put, if the mind is positive, the body will have the best chance to achieve challenges. On the other hand, if the body is positive about meeting a challenge, the mind will support the body in achieving the challenge.

Experts say that the mind produces more than fifty thousand thoughts daily. They say that the mind constantly thinks of and chats about things from the past or what might happen in the future, not bothering much with what might be happening in the present moment. One day I counted seventy-five different thoughts my mind skimmed across in a matter of only two minutes. On and on and on it thought, filling my head with past things not worth remembering or future things not worth worrying about.

"Today, we accept that there is a powerful mind–body connection through which emotional, mental, social, spiritual, and behavioral factors can directly affect our health," says the National Institutes of Health (National Institutes of Health 2008) Other experts agree that a communication link between the mind and body occurs in the form of nerve impulses in the brain, which turns on biochemical reactions in the body. We have all had this communication link since birth, even if we have not realized it. Feeling butterflies in the stomach when approaching the podium to make a speech, salivating at the thought or the sight of a favorite desert, or feeling nervous when meeting a favorite movie star are all examples of the mind's influence over the body's reactions.

Another example that has most likely happened to all of us is waking up from a bad dream with your heart racing (due to an electrical reaction turned on by the mind) and body drenched in sweat (due to a chemical reaction turned on by the mind). Your mind experienced the dream as real and reacted by releasing biochemical and electrical reactions in your body—even though you were sound asleep and had no clue about what was happening in your mind or body. Your mind was aware, which turned on your body's reaction. In turn, your body's reaction woke you up.

These are simple but real examples of how the mind can transform thoughts and feelings into chemical and electrical impulses and send them to the body, causing your body to react. In other words, the reaction is the way your body responds to what is happening in your mind. This process happens nearly instantaneously. Remember, we also have a body–mind communication connection. If you pay close attention, you will see the impact the body has on the mind. An example of a body–mind reaction is the common cold. Often people begin to feel "not themselves" a few days before the sniffles, sore throat, or other common symptoms appear. Also, the body can convince the mind to approach a challenge in a positive manner, where the mind in turn reacts by causing the body to react in biochemical or electrical ways.

Kulreet Chaudhary, MD, a pioneer in the field of integrative medicine says:

> If we are constantly thinking negative, self-destructive thoughts, our bodies will follow suit. Emotional and mental imbalance can start as something like stress-induced headaches, tight shoulders, and a sore upper back and lead to unhealthy weight gain or loss, insomnia, and high blood pressure. On the other hand, we can make a conscious effort to think more positively and to develop healthy coping mechanisms for life's stresses and trials. Over time, the state of our emotional and mental health can hurt or help the body's immune system.
>
> We can make ourselves sick and we can make ourselves well. Studies show our coping mechanisms and ways we handle stress directly correlate to how we deal with serious illnesses, including cancer. Chronic stress affects the body in a negative way, and over long periods of time, long-term stress can make us more susceptible to diabetes, hypertension, heart diseases, and some infections. However, by using our innate mind–body connection in a positive way, by keeping our minds and bodies in shape with exercise and nutrition, we can keep stress levels lower. In other words, the better we can cope by staying calm and reducing psychological stress, we will in-turn reduce physical stress, along with the chance of developing a disease. (Chaudhary 2016)

I've come up with another adage that could have been coined at the same time as the "We are what we eat" adage: "We are what we eat and how much we move." Experts agree that today a sedentary life is the new smoking. Moving your body moves your mind to release endorphins in the body that reduce psychological stress, which in turn reduces physical stress levels. Research shows that keeping the mind and body healthy through exercise and nutrition can ward off certain diseases and conditions. It can also set up the conditions to think positive as a lifestyle habit.

We should be aware, however, that sometimes the mind–body communication link could produce negative outcomes, like failing to meet goals that we have worked extra hard to achieve. For some time, my mind had a tendency toward negative thoughts about some of my challenges. My first year at my new high school is a case in point. This kind of negative thinking is commonly referred to in the mind–body field as automatic negative thoughts, or ANT. As the term implies, my negative thoughts were happening so habitually that I did not realize that they were seriously minimizing my chances of achieving even my most simple challenge.

One challenge that plagued me for many months dealt with running. My mind had been telling me for years that I was not fast enough to run the gold standard of marathons in the USA: the Boston Marathon. Because the Boston race course has a hilly second half, topped off at about mile twenty by Heartbreak Hill, I included a similar hill in my morning six-mile training run. I told myself that I had to run nonstop to the top of my quarter-mile hill to manage

Heartbreak Hill. Each morning during my training run, my mindset was so resolute that my body would begin to falter before I got to within five hundred feet of that hill. I had been engaging in hard hill training for months. I did not realize it at the time, but my body could run that hill nonstop—my mind did not know that my body could.

One day I said to myself, "You have been training for months on hills and have proven your proficiency on many other hills. What's with this hill? Is it because it mimics Heartbreak Hill? Is it about stress?" That was when I began to practice deeper breathing before my hill came into view. Somehow, breathing deeply made the hill less menacing; although at the time I still could not make it to the top without walking. Each day I continued the deeper breathing, which I appropriately named the One Breath Focus, because that's what I did: I focused on only one breath at a time. One Breath Focus minimizes the mind's tendency to employ ANT because the technique keeps the mind busy focusing on the pathways the air takes on inhale and exhale.

By constantly using the One Breath Focus technique of breathing, the power of the mind's chatter weakened as the mind's chatter diminished considerably. As a result, this breathing technique became my routine way of breathing. With a quiet mind, I could more easily focus it on the positive. I would simply think of the passion I felt when I could not respond to my three-year-old in her original game of tag earlier. I simply compare my health status then with my present state of health. So when I hear the whining voice of an unsettled, negative mind, I pause and use the One Breath Focus technique.

What I uncovered in this process was a simple two-step technique that has been working for me for years, changing my mind and body mindsets from negative to positive. I named the technique Positive Linkups, or PLUS. It consists of (1) establishing and maintaining excellent posture for effective deep breathing and (2) carrying out the One Breath Focus technique. This technique is nature-based in that good posture will be achieved by reaching your hands way up to the sky, which stacks one vertebra in your back on top of the other, from the base of your head to your tail bone. In addition, position your ears over your shoulders while simultaneously positioning your chin parallel to the ground. Great posture allows your lungs and diaphragm to participate more easily in very deep breathing. And focusing on deep breathing tends to quiet the mind which, in turn, allows for more intense focusing as you move your mind and/or your body from negative to positive thinking. The PLUS lifestyle takes you from a glass half-full lifestyle to a glass running-over lifestyle. As a result, PLUS became my blueprint for living; it's positive zest added zing to life as it deposited a better chance of meeting life's challenges right in my own two hands.

PLUS, could become your blueprint for living, but it will not be easy, especially if you have been drowning in the agony of ANTs because of so many failed diet-type attempts at becoming healthier. Despite my ten years of fitness and nutrition failed attempts running with the diet herd, I made a complete turnaround from ANTs to PLUS.

⚠ You must keep pushing harder today than you pushed yesterday to guarantee healthier tomorrows. It takes a wealth of butterfly-type patience and dandelion-type passionverance to successfully reap healthier lifestyle outcomes for the rest of your life. Remember. Using nature's principles of patience and passionverance will allow you to expertly internalize the important information presented in this section. Know that the information presented here becomes the core of the next step in the process. It is also important to note that at each step you are gradually required to be yourself in this process.

Part 3

Step Three of Nature's Six-Step Formula: Nutrition and Movement Harmony

Simply stated, every time you eat junk or nutritious food, sit still or move actively, you are either feeding disease or fighting disease.

—B. H. Smith

Passionverance opens the doors to step three of nature's six-step formula: nutrition and movement harmony. A major part of sealing in lifestyle changes is through your nutrition and movement activities. Scientific research outcomes are adamant about how critical proper nutrients and movement activities are to minimize certain diseases and conditions, as well as helping to slow the aging process. Good nutrition is critical for renewing dead cells with healthier cells, and movement activities are critical for those renewed cells to come back strong, flexible, balanced, and relaxed.

A truly wise person said that true healthcare reform begins in your kitchen, not in Washington, DC. And my five siblings and I learned all that we needed to know about true health and other essentials about life at our kitchen table—the only space in our house that could accommodate six children and our parents. The significance of harmony within nature's six-step formula reminds me of my parents' weekly kitchen table routine, which could have been called Holston family harmony. In a regular ritual spearheaded by our father, all six of us kids were actively taught to live together in harmony.

Most Saturday evenings after dinner, Daddy would ask one of us to bring him the broom. Back then, brooms were made of individual straw pieces, which could be pulled apart. He would individually pull eight straws from the broom and place them on the table just in front of him. He would count each straw piece. He would then pick up one straw and easily break it in half. He would pass the next straw to mother at the other end of the table. He would ask her to break it in half as well. He would pass a single straw to each of the rest of us and ask each of us to break them. Each of us complied until we all had single broken straws in front of us. Daddy would then pull eight new straws from the broom and bind them together by twisting. He would pass the twisted straws around to mother and ask her to try to break the group of twisted straws. Mother would try to break them, but of course she could not. Each child got the chance to try to break the eight twisted straws. Of course, no one could. Daddy would say, "We are one family in harmony, just like this cluster of eight straws. When we stick together as a family like these straws, we will remain in harmony as a family and nothing can ever weaken any one of us."

That is the same point that nature teaches about her cluster of two straws, called nutrition and fitness. Good nutrition without active movement or active movement without good nutrition leads to weaker new cells, which means a less healthy body over time.

And it is the same nutrition and movement harmony message that the late Dr. Lodge and co-author Christopher Crowley saluted in their book *Younger Next Year*. Dr. Lodge was interested in primary care and preventive medicine, and was deeply committed to the role of healthy lifestyle in medical care. (Lodge and Crowley 2007)

Most aging is just the dry rot we program into our cells by sedentary living, junk food and stress. You replace about 1 percent of your cells every day. That means 1 percent of your body is brand new today, and you will get another 1 percent tomorrow. Think of it as getting a whole new body, every three months. It's not entirely accurate, but it's pretty close. Viewed that way, you are walking around in a body that is brand new after three months. Whether that body is functionally younger or older is a choice you make by how you live.

I decided to consider replacing my old cells every day with cells that were the strongest possible. Albert Einstein led the way for me. He said that it makes no sense to believe that you will get different results by continuing to do the same things that resulted in the situation that you wish to change. In other words, Einstein was saying that change was in order. My mind and body needed to work in harmony to support strengthening my new cells, rather than replacing dying cells with new but weaker cells. I began to gradually make routine changes to the likes of eating fresh, raw blueberries that strengthen cells rather than blueberry pie a la mode, which weakens them, and walking outside after dinner rather than watching TV. As a result, I began to gradually harmonize eating good nutritious food with daily active exercise.

I had to begin to take full advantage of my living inside of nature. My mind told me that I only had access to the nutrition and movement activities that nature would approve. I believed my mind, that sitting on the couch, watching TV and eating blueberry pie was not to be had anywhere inside nature's world. All I needed to do was to have my body follow through.

It worked. Since both good nutrition and active movement activities are like identical twins in nature's cluster of two twisted straws, my own cluster of those two straws were so connected that I could not think of nutrition without also thinking of active movement activities, and vice versa. One could say that it became a single-minded focus on one swallow for good nutrition and one breath for active fitness activities. That is how the phrase "one swallow, one breath" stuck in my mind and eventually became my mantra.

My bottom line on nutrition and movement is that the body is by far the most complex machine on earth, more complex than anything made by humans. Although complex, the body can be tended to according to nature's most simplistic ways to keep it strong, flexible, balanced, and relaxed, even as it ages.

As I was striving to improve my nutrition and fitness habits in the simplest ways possible, a bright light went off in my head. I knew that I needed to figure out not only how to love replacing old cells with new healthy cells, but to also love the activities it would take to do so. Through steadfast thinking I realized that nature had already programmed into the process her simple answer: we humans must eliminate emotional eating and emotional fitness from our lives and replace them with functional eating and functional fitness. When considered through nature's eyes, emotional eating and emotional fitness had nothing to do with becoming healthy because they catered to everything outside of the needs of keeping the body as healthy as possible. For example, whenever emotions are involved, the focus is on making sure that there is a winning outcome no matter what. (Winning outcomes for emotional eating might be, "Does it taste good?" or "Can I still eat my deep-fried chicken or rare steaks?" Winning outcomes for emotional fitness might be, "Do I have to give up my favorite ten hours a day of TV programs?" or "Can I text while walking with a purpose?") Whenever functions are involved, the focus is on making sure that the body has all that it needs for developing strong replacement cells, and functioning like a well oil machine.

This simple emotion–function process has helped me focus on eating right and moving actively. But I needed to learn the ins and outs of good nutrition and active movement. What do I eat for optimal nutrition, and how do I move for optimal fitness? Since there was scarce information available in the popular media so many years ago, I turned back to nature and to my forward-thinking board-certified Dr. Mirkin's radio show for trusted answers.

Functional Nutrition

Years before medical science joined the nutrition/wellness bandwagon, Dr. Mirkin recommended eating a variety of fruits, vegetables, whole grains, beans, seeds, and nuts and cutting back on animal protein. Similarly, this food selection is what nature would want for a healthy body and mind. (Mirkin 2014). I added to Dr. Mirkin's advice. Over time, I not only cut back on animal protein but deleted it completely from my life. As my youngest brother used to say, "I don't eat anything that has a face." Later, I also excluded all conventionally grown food, in favor of certified organic foods. One could say that after I moved inside nature, her influence on my lifestyle was relentless.

These drastic changes in my eating and moving habits came not without hours of seeking out information and educating myself. Over more than thirty years, I used research outcomes reported by Dr. Mirkin on his show and later when research outcomes were reported by research universities and others in lay newsletters. From these sources, I had access to a whole host of credible expert organizations and individuals to make sure that my body had access to all that it needed to remain healthy and constantly replace dying cells with stronger versions. It was my passion for knowledge about good nutrition and healthy movement activities that drove me from within to scrutinize and vigorously digest information from all credible sources that I could get my hands on. Over time, I studied hundreds and hundreds of reports on research outcomes from nationally respected nutrition and movement experts:

- University research newsletters (such as from the University of California, Harvard, Tufts, Johns Hopkins, and Duke, and health newsletters such as *Environmental Nutrition*, Dr. Gabe Mirkin's *Mirkin Report Newsletter* and Mirkin's online *E-Zine Fitness*

and Health Newsletter, The Mount Sinai Healthy Aging Newsletter; and others)
- Health, fitness, and nutrition gurus (such as Dr. Gabe Mirkin of Kensington, Maryland; the Mid-Atlantic Region's Kaiser Permanente medical staff; AARP, and others)
- Food/health advocate organizations (such as the Center for Science in the Public Interest, American Association of Retired Persons, American Cancer Society, and others)
- The federal government and professional organizations and clinics (such as the National Institutes of Health, the US Department of Agriculture, Center for Disease Control and Prevention, American Cancer Society, the Cleveland and Mayo Clinics, and others)
- Health columns (such as from *Time Magazine*, the *New York Times*, the *Washington Post*, and others)

I was very much influenced by an article that appeared in the Tufts University Health & Nutrition Letter special supplement; the headline read "Eating to Beat Cancer— *Experts blame one-third of all cancers on diet and lifestyle. But cutting-edge research suggests some foods may help prevent cancer."* When the doctors at Harvard Medical School were asked, 'Do natural cancer-fighters exist?' The response was, 'Yes. So far, it is generally accepted that ginger, green tea, and pomegranates contain natural cancer inhibitors." (Tufts University Health & Nutrition Letter, 2007). Headlines such as this are only the tip of the food/

disease research iceberg. Science constantly highlights findings such as these because of ongoing research.

The information that I absorbed seemed to automatically cluster into three categories. Each category was of equal importance to overall health. One category without the other two was not as effective. Each category is as important as each leg of a three-leg stool is to the functionality of the stool. The first category, nutrients, includes water soluble vitamins, fat soluble vitamins, antioxidants, macronutrient minerals, and micronutrient minerals. The second category, food types, includes high-quality whole fruits, vegetables, whole grains, dried beans, seeds, and nuts, along with distilled water for drinking and cooking. The third category, good for you features, includes foods that are organic, high in fiber, plant-based, and vegan, and foods that contain low monounsaturated and polyunsaturated fats, complex carbohydrates, and low sodium.

Nutrition experts are adamant that once digested, the three categories do their work in the body by eventually making high-quality nutrient deposits directly in the blood. The Mayo Clinic says that your body is a battleground against infections and diseases because it uses wholesome blood to replace cells that have died. In other words, this process clears the way to allow your body to function more healthfully and efficiently.

To make this wealth of nutrient information easier to use, I arranged it according to a three-column matrix that includes the name of the nutrient in column one, the nutrient's best food sources in column two, and the nutrient's health possibilities in column three. Health possibilities are gleamed from respected scientific research outcomes. The chart, called Nature's Nourishment, is available in Appendix A.

Thankfully, nature has a standard way of organizing her operations, which gives us the opportunity to understand and best use nature's wisdom. To better organize lifestyle change operations in keeping with nature's orderly ways, I developed a standard way of sticking to my new nutritious lifestyle. I generated a set of guidelines based on my years following and emulating nature. These guidelines are made up of sets of principles, properties, food categories, daily essential foods, serving choices, and grazing times.

- Principles: ego management, open to change, risk taking, thriving on pressure, and goal-oriented

These qualities of success principles, when banded together like that cluster of straws, grant great potential for handling change in an intelligent manner. The late Stephen Hawkings reminded us that, "Intelligence is the ability to adapt to change." Therefore, these principles provide help in adapting to changing lifelong unhealthy habits in favor of new nutritious habits. For many, the ego seems to hamper progress by putting itself front and center for most things in life. The principle of ego management allowed me to know that the ego might be an impediment. I moved my ego completely out of my way as I worked to change my eating ways. The principle of being open to change is a constant green light to see change through to victory. The principle of risk taking comes with the expectation to constantly "stick the neck out," as you continue making progress to victory. Without the principle of thriving on pressure, you might become weary and throw in the towel before victory. The principle of being goal-oriented helps you remain focused on the prize, no matter what blocks your path.

- Properties: vegan foods, organic foods, whole foods, complex carbohydrates, olive oil, low-fat foods, high-fiber foods, 50/50 raw/cooked, cooked foods are prepared in water at 212 degrees or less.

This powerful grouping clustered together is a sample of properties that form the most nutritious base possible for the highest quality nutrition achievable. The highest quality nutrition is simply not possible if the base is lacking in any one of these critical properties.

- Food categories: carbohydrates, protein, and fats

Complex carbohydrates instead of simple carbohydrates, vegetable-based protein instead of animal protein, and monounsaturated/polyunsaturated fat instead of saturated fat are the hallmarks of what the body needs to have the best chance for replacing cells with strong, healthy new cells.

- Daily essential foods: fruits, vegetables, whole grains, dried beans, seeds, nuts, and distilled water

You must have foods from each of these food groups (plus water) each day to make sure that you eat a variety of foods in response to the recommend daily allowance, as recommended by government nutrition experts. Selecting foods from each category assumes that the body follows an anti-inflammatory lifestyle as it receives all the nutrients possible to build strong, healthy new cells. Include a wide variety of colors every day as extra insurance. Distilled water is made up of two parts oxygen and one-part hydrogen and is extra insurance that chemicals used by governments to purify water are not what nature would recommend. Specific daily essential foods: celery, curry, garlic, onion, ginger, chia seeds, banana, green tea, walnuts, broccoli, and blueberries are foods known to science as super foods and are included in my daily eating patterns as extra insurance. You might note that processed and unprocessed animal protein has been totally removed from my eating plan over 30 years ago because of ongoing research outcomes that showed "increased rates of death from cancer, heart disease, stroke, diabetes, respiratory disease, infections, kidney disease and liver disease." (Mirkin 2007)

- Serving choices: broth, loaf, soup, stew, and unblended whole foods

An assortment of serving choices provides variety to keep meals attention-grabbing, appealing, interesting, and exciting.

- Grazing times: breakfast, midmorning mini snack, lunch, afternoon mini snack, dinner, early evening mini snack.

Grazing provides opportunity to ingest smaller meals throughout the day and early evening. Experts seem to agree that eating smaller meals over the course of the day is more beneficial than the customary three meals. Experts also tend to recommend eating the heaviest meals early on and eating lighter meals as the day progresses.

After I followed nature's wisdom and categorized my eating ways into emotional and functional eating, along with using "Nature's Nourishment" chart (Appendix A), it was a no brainer to just say yes to foods that function healthily in the body and no to foods that function unhealthily in the body. I remember making the easy choice by saying to myself, "Which side is this food on: the healthy side or the unhealthy side?" Over time, I deleted all emotional eating from my lifestyle.

Following is a true story about how changing nutrition habits for the better impacted one family's life. My friend's husband at one point went kicking and screaming from emotional eating to functional eating. As a result, the heart attack that he had when he was mid-stream into letting go of emotional eating and replacing it with functional eating (and walking) saved his life, according to his doctors. He began as obese, middle-aged, out of shape, easy-chair, TV-clicker. He had lifestyle-driven high blood pressure and was prediabetic (most likely due to his emotional eating lifestyle). His wife was worried about his health. She had heard about my eating for health and asked me to give her some of my recipes. She thought that maybe she could convince her husband to give up some of his red meat and potatoes with lots of butter and sour cream, which he dearly loved, for a few vegetables every now and then.

I told my friend that my way of making sure that I included all the vitamins and minerals that my body needed was not based on a bunch of recipes, but a bunch of ingredients from which I make my own recipes, tailored to my own health needs and tastes. She could select ingredients for her own recipes according to her and her husband's individual health needs and tastes. The ingredients I selected for my new eating lifestyle should be ingested regularly to give the body exactly what it needs to replace old cells with new cells which are healthy and strong. I gave my friend a copy of my "Nature's Nourishment" charts (Appendix A). As she looked them over, she asked, "How do I use these charts?"

I explained to my friend that in keeping with nature's rules of simplicity, the charts in Appendix A are organized for easy use. First, in column one, I broke down vitamins and minerals into four main categories: water-soluble vitamins, fat-soluble vitamins, antioxidants and macro/micro minerals. In column two, for each category, a listing of associated foods is provided. In column three, for each category, a listing of associated science-based major health possibilities is provided. I use the charts not only for meal planning, which I individualize to my own likes and taste, I also use them to attack health issues I may need to address. Finally I use the information to build my recipes, menus, and shopping lists.

For example, let's look at the antioxidant beta-carotene that's included in column one under the heading "Antioxidants." The best food sources for beta-carotene according to studies are orange, yellow, and dark green fruits and vegetables. In column three under beta-carotene are health possibilities that highlight how the antioxidant helps prevent night blindness and age-related macular degeneration; it may also protect against certain types of cancer.

At your fingertips is a listing of food sources, such as carrots, sweet potatoes, kale, and spinach, to include beta-carotene in meal planning. A hearty meal can be served that includes kale, sweet potatoes, added mushrooms, and whole grains and seeds, along with a green salad. Or I might pick and choose other foods that represent a variety of colors and make a chia seed/mushroom/vegetable loaf, stew, or soup. Your bottom line is that you select foods that you and your husband adore which are based on health possibilities that are important to you. At the same time, the big bonus is that you will replace old cells with strong, healthy cells.

I cautioned my friend to make sure that her husband checked in with his doctor before changing anything, and then I directed her to look down the "Health Possibilities" column in the chart to find which nutrients science believes will help reduce high blood pressure or prevent it from rising. The next step would be to make a shopping list of the corresponding best food sources. And finally, after collecting the needed ingredients, make an "anti-high blood pressure" meal and serve it as a stew, broth, loaf, soup, or unblended food plate.

My friend followed through and served her husband a vegetable/mushroom/whole grain stew, but she forgot to include his super-hot peppers, which he dearly loves. He took one taste and his emotionally driven taste buds yelled, "Yuck!" Although his long years of emotional eating for taste got him into trouble with his health, he simply did not care. He, like so many others, made emotionally driven taste a higher priority than functionally driven well-being. His wife figured out what to do to help him switch from emotions to functions: she sprinkled hot peppers on the stew. He ate the whole bowl and went back for seconds. Later, she told me about his forceful reaction to the new dish. In their household the new eating lifestyle became formally known as the "Yuck Eating Lifestyle" or "Yuck."

Since that time, my friend has "jazzed" up Yuck with hot peppers and all types of healthy spices and herbs that she and her husband adore. It made the difference. She would make great batches of Yuck and freeze individual servings as loafs, soups, or stews. She was so proud that she could have healthy meals in a flash for weeks at a time. Instead of stopping on the way home to buy fast food, she goes straight home, opens her freezer and have "fast food" in a flash. Over time, her husband gradually changed his eating habits. It has been years since that first outing with Yuck, and they eat versions of Yuck for most meals. He has dropped nearly a third of his weight, has moderated his blood pressure and cholesterol, is no longer prediabetic, and is now a serious walker, walking well over twenty-five hours weekly.

A couple years after his first encounter with Yuck, my friend's husband woke up one morning not feeling well enough to get out the door with gusto to greet the sun for his morning walk. He felt worse by midday. He went to see his doctor. He was taken almost immediately to surgery, where he received a triple by-pass operation. His doctor told him that his life was saved because of the changes he made in his eating and moving lifestyle— losing eighty pounds eating Yuck and walking daily. He had changed his lifestyle just in the nick of time. As a result, he was up on his feet and walking just hours after his surgery.

Today, if he were asked to come up with a name for this new way of eating, he would still call this functional partner to aerobic movement, Yuck. For him Yuck now stands for yams, unsaturated fat, chia seeds, and kale. All these things are powerhouse ingredients that mean high-quality, plant-based complete protein, heart-friendly mono-unsaturated fat, and antioxidant-dense complex carbohydrates. This makes for a meal that uses whole foods and is balanced, low fat, low sodium, plant-based, and delicious.

The beauty of the Yuck eating lifestyle is that it can be tailored to individual taste and can provide an assortment of food and serving choices. Most of all, you do not have to feel deprived and you never have to go to bed hungry or unsatisfied! All you need to do is to make sure that all ingredients fit within nature's wisdom on functional eating. So, go ahead and select your favorite fruits, vegetables, whole grains, dried beans, seeds, and nuts from the list in

Appendix A and jazz your selections up with the spices and herbs of your choice. Based on the latest of all that science knows about the benefits to health of good nutrition, we are not about diets here. We favor an eating lifestyle that has the very best opportunity to bring back strong, healthier cells rather than weak, unhealthy cells. Just think—you can forever stamp out yo-yo diets because you can eat the functional lifestyle way for the rest of your life.

Functional Movement

Here is another true story, but this time it is about how I fell into functional movement and how it became a regular part of my life. For those unfamiliar, let me share some information about how the body functions. I read an article years ago, but the piece didn't speak to me back then as it did in 2007. I was jerked upright by the late Dr. Henry S. Lodge's inflamed voice on the pages of an article published in Parade Magazine section of the Washington Post. (Parade Magazine 2007). It was as if Lodge was right there in my head. Lodge's words were yelling about movement. The titles and subtitles from the *Parade Magazine* article that first got my undivided attention were "You can stop 'normal' aging," "Most aging is just the dry rot we program into our cells by sedentary living, junk food, and stress," and "You can stop 'normal' aging if you are willing to do the work." "Dry" and "rot"—I was surely ready to continue to do the hard work. Lodge more than makes the case for fitness. In fact, he took the words right out of my mouth and plastered them in the magazine for the world to read.

Lodge's words take interested people by the shoulders and shake them awake. In the article, he summarized his research appealing to lay people like me. He told why fitness is so important to the aging body. He told us exactly how the human body responds to the way we treat it day in and day out. He let us know in plain English that a sedentary lifestyle wreaks daily havoc in some way or another on each cell in our bodies. And he said all of it in the most powerful way that I have ever read from any source.

The Mayo Clinic and Mirkin, among many other experts, deliver the same message as Lodge. The Mayo staff talked openly about how beneficial exercise is to health and well-being. They asked, "We all know that exercise is good for us. But do we know just how good?" Mayo Clinic staff answered their own question:

> You can feel better, add more years to your life and at the same time have much more energy. The health benefits of regular exercise and physical activity are hard to ignore. Everyone benefits from exercise, regardless of age, sex, or physical ability. Constant exercise controls weight, combats health conditions and diseases, improves mood. Regular exercise helps prevent or manage a wide range of health problems and concerns, including stroke, metabolic syndrome, type 2 diabetes and depression, a number of types of cancer, arthritis and falls. And it boosts energy as well. (Mayo Clinic 2016).

"When the body is conditioned," said the late Dr. George Sheehan, one of my running heroes, "running is like being the full orchestra, which has been brought alive by the spirit of the conductor." (Sheehan 1989). Nature stands on the podium and taps her baton to alert (the human body) her orchestra that the concert is about to begin. Nature's spirit—balanced, flexible, relaxed, and strong—stands ready to function as one with the members of her orchestra. Her orchestra is a self-contained masterpiece of engineering systems, which includes a central control center, message signaling, warming and cooling systems, a breathing apparatus, fighting marines, an exchange procedure, a food processor, a waste disposal, a reproduction technique, a sensory scheme, a motor system, hinges, pumps, levers, factories, fibers, and an elastic, waterproof coating to keep all systems in place, safe and sound inside. This orchestra of body parts is more complex than anything created by humans on earth. Although complex, however, it requires the simplest, most uncomplicated levels of support to keep it running smoothly.

Successful functioning is guaranteed with nature at the helm. Everything is done in harmony, from the fuel the body needs for good health to how the body was designed to move. Every instrument is strong, flexible, balanced, and relaxed in ways that nature stipulates. Nature leaves you breathless with her music without an off-beat or missed note.

On the other hand, if you use any part of your body in ways that nature did not design for its use, things can go very wrong. For example, if you smoke, you might get lung cancer or heart disease problems. If you overeat or eat the wrong things, you might get heart disease problems or become obese, which can set you up for type 2 diabetes and certain cancers. If you are sedentary, you might get type 2 diabetes, hypertension, heart disease problems, or certain cancers. If you eat too much red meat, you might get kidney disease problems.

Because of Lodge, Mirkin, the Mayo Clinic, and many other experts, I had more respect for the movement activities that I had been engaged in for years. After reading Dr. Lodge's "dry rot" quote, my movement activities took on a more important tone. I intensified my morning routine to make sure that I was doing the strengthening, flexibility, balance, and relaxation activities vigorously enough. I also had more awareness of the number of weekly miles that I was running. I wanted to make sure that I was running enough miles to count in improving my replacement cells.

After beginning the changes to my lifestyle, I read the following from Dr. Lodge: "When we exercise, that process of growth spreads throughout every cell in our bodies, making us functionally younger. Not a little bit younger—a lot younger." I was more adamant than ever to make sure that I was right on target with my entire lifestyle. I know that it is very difficult to exercise routinely, but if it is a part of your lifestyle, it is something you end up doing almost as automatically as breathing.

According to most experts, your passionverance for movement can be walking, jogging, running, but it must be weight bearing to focus on keeping the bones strong and healthy. The President's Council on Fitness, Sports &

Nutrition says that bone-strengthening exercises produce a force on the bones that promotes bone growth and strength. This force is commonly produced by impact with the ground. (President's Council on Fitness, Sports & Nutrition n.d.)

To keep the heart as strong as possible as you age, you can bike, row, or engage in other non–weight bearing exercises. Remember, for heart fitness, keep moving for a minimum of thirty minutes without stopping to elevate your heart rate up twenty beats above its resting rate; keep it there for at least thirty minutes without stopping. Do this most days of the week.

After I categorized my lifestyle program activities into emotional and functional categories, it was a no brainer to just say yes to functional fitness activities and no to any emotional ego-driven activity. I remember making the easy choice by saying to myself, "Which side is this activity on: the healthy side or the unhealthy side?" Over time, I deleted all emotionally driven lifestyle activities that were within my power to delete. That's when I began to sail along life like an ageless sensation.

It is said by the majority of health-conscious scientist that nutrition and fitness are on equal footing when it comes to replacing cells in the healthiest ways possible. And that cluster of two straws, nutrition and fitness, says ingesting food—even nutritious food—is not enough alone to become optimally healthy. I learned this fact the hard way after running with the diet herd for at least ten years.

Nancy S. Mure (Mure n.d.) said, "Obesity is not a disease. It is a lifestyle affliction. It is a symptom. It is a side effect of poor habits and it can be reversed."

Mure was right. I began to go outside to walk, and then gradually I began to run. Back in the late 1960s and early 1970s, if people were walking or running at all, most were going from point A to point B, not because of fitness.

Before beginning any exercise program, I suggest that you do what I did to remain injury-free. First, check in with and get an okay from your healthcare professionals. Second, ready your posture by exercising your body in the areas of strength, flexibility, balance, and relaxation. These enrichment exercises will help you establish a baseline upon which to build your entire functional fitness program. (See Appendix B: Alignment)

Come with me, way back to when I first began making the fitness change from an out-of-shape, overweight, junk-food loving, sedentary person to the fit, ultra-marathon runner that I am today, in my seventh decade of life. "What in the world are you doing out there in sweat pants, an old T-shirt- and your worn-out tennis shoes? You look a mess! Neighbors will think that you are 'touched' in the head or something." These are the kind of comments that I got from family, friends, and others who I did not even know. But those comments did not deter me. I was on a mission of function. My ego was left inside, in the back, in the corner, in the dark, way out of sight.

Functional eating and functional fitness reflect upon one of nature's greatest laws because together they round out best opportunities to replace dying cells. Over the years I continuously updated both the nutrition and the fitness information in response to updates in the medical research. I have remained so totally on track that my immune system is super strong. I have had no aches, pains, colds or flu in more than three decades. Each morning I'm filled with energy and ready to take on whatever life brings. I end my ultra-marathons with more energy than when I began. My heart is so strong that my pulse rate varies between 28 to 32 beats per minute on rest and up to a maximum of 135 beats per minute during near anaerobic running. My blood pressure hovers around 106/68. My good cholesterol (HDL) is never lower than 77 mg/dL. My glucose post-fast hovers around 88 mg/dL and my triglycerides hover around 41 mg/dL. At age seventy-one, my femur bone density showed thickening rather than thinning. The results of a university research study that I participated in more than a dozen years ago concluded that my vital statistics were that of a healthy twenty-five-year-old. I was about sixty-one years old at the time.

⚠️ You must keep pushing harder today than you pushed yesterday to guarantee healthier tomorrows. It takes a wealth of butterfly-type patience and dandelion-type passionverance to successfully reap healthier lifestyle outcomes for the rest of your life. Remember. Using nature's principles of patience and passionverance will allow you to expertly internalize the important information presented in this section. Know that the information presented here becomes the core of the next step in the process. It is also important to note that at each step you are gradually required to be yourself in this process.

> We do not stop exercising because we grow old; we grow old because we stop exercising.
>
> —Dr. Kenneth Cooper

Part 3

Step Four of Nature's Six-Step Formula: Lifestyle Change Line

And the day came when the risk to remain tight in a bud was more painful than the risk it took to blossom.

—Anais Nin

And blossom I did. Just like that dandelion, I did the hard work to rise out of the cement to greet the rays of the sunshine. Now passionverance's rewards await me with open arms.

Passionverance opens the doors to step four of nature's six-step formula: lifestyle change line. Passionverance eventually pushes you—sometimes kicking and screaming—over the lifestyle change line. You reach the line only if you have taken steps one, two and three to heart. After you cross the line, your struggles disappear. Your mind relaxes. Your mind and body want you to continue your nutrition and movement activities. You are settled into your new lifestyle. This means that the new you is your new lifestyle.

When I think of what dandelions have accomplished, since they have been around for centuries and are able to bloom brightly out of a crack in the sidewalk, I see the dandelion's passionverance as tantamount to my own passionverance. It is in response to my struggle to make it up to and across the lifestyle change line. Once across the line, nature's secret support system showered me with gifts.

I made it through step one of the lifestyle change system's six-step formula, where I tapped into my internal strength. I called upon my internal strength repeatedly to wade through the shoulder-high water of step two, mind–body harmony.

Steps one and two prepared me to completely change my nutrition and fitness habits as my body and mind wrestled through step three, nutrition and fitness harmony. Some experiences in life are so intimate, so deep that they defy description, because they can only be experienced, not described. I had no words to describe the experience when I first stepped across the lifestyle change line at step four.

I imagined that the mysterious quality of my line-crossing experience must have been like the experience of a new mother glimpsing her first newborn, just moments after birth, or Armstrong's first step on the moon—experiences that go way beyond words. The moment I realized that my line crossing put me into a very different realm of eating and moving was so personal and intimate that it could not even be understood by others until they stepped across themselves.

Earl Nightingale once declared, "Whatever we plant in our subconscious mind and nourish with repetition and emotion will one day become our reality." (Nightingale n.d.) I know that I repeatedly told myself that I should only eat or move in ways sanctioned by nature. I knew that I had progressively made many conscious nutrition and fitness attempts at changes for the healthier throughout steps one through three. While in the process, I had no idea that my subconscious mind was working hard to gradually take over my eating and fitness choices.

Nature's support system kicked in the moment that I crossed the line. I have no scientific backup for thinking that the most important segment of nature's support system is housed in the subconscious mind. My subconscious mind was activated the moment I crossed the line. I believed that I had internalized nature's wisdom on eating and moving at the subconscious level because I suddenly was able to follow nature's wisdom as automatically as the heart beats. Suddenly my relationship with eating my favorite unhealthy food, such as the entire homemade German chocolate cake, was the same as my desire to eat dirt crawling with worms! In addition, I was no longer tempted to eat foods that would contribute to my ill health. Also, I made no judgments about the foods that others ate.

My mind's focus was on eating and moving like never before. The center of attention was wholly on fighting diseases or conditions, not augmenting diseases or conditions. Although I had no words to describe it, the evidence was crystal clear: I had indeed made subconscious changes and nature's reward was a support system housed in my subconscious mind. Nature's steadfast support system only allowed nutrition and fitness activities that are sanctioned by nature. Therefore, I no longer had a desire for unhealthy foods or non-movement activities, which contributed to building weaker replacement cells. My complete turnaround had nothing to do with the level of discipline that it took for me to take step one. It was nature's support system, which was turned on in and managed by my subconscious mind.

Before crossing the line, back when I had to muster all the discipline inside of myself to follow nature's commands, family and friends did not have a clue about nature's rewards. In fact, some believed that I was obsessed. For example, early on, when I attempted to eat nutritiously, family members, colleagues, and friends at the table at the time ordered their customary meals. Instead of ordering my normal high-calorie, highly processed, unhealthy meal, I ordered a simple salad and planned to fortify it with my own salad dressing and chickpeas brought from home. Based on their reactions, you would have thought that I pulled a live rabbit from my tote bag to eat right there at the lunch table.

When I went to Paris and London with my running friends to run the Paris and London marathons a week apart, I filled one suitcase with small cans of chickpeas, enough for two weeks of protein. I figured that I could order a salad or other vegetable to round out my meals. To me, my lifestyle was every moment, so it did not differ because I was in Paris or London with the opportunity to pig out on high-calorie, high-fat, low-fiber foods. My running friends told me that my lifestyle should not matter. After all, I was in places that were world famous for their wine, cheese, bread, and other cuisine. They were amazed that I was satisfied with the chickpeas and green vegetables that I ate throughout my time there. Toward the end of the trip, one runner, who had ingested probably seven thousand calories each day, told me that I was the most disciplined person he had ever known. "How could you deprive yourself in such a manner? You never deviated to eat one luscious meal," he said. I responded by telling him that my lifestyle is every moment. He had no clue that it meant that it took much less discipline when you are nearing the lifestyle change line.

Another instance that comes to mind is one that really got my running friends talking about my zany ways. It was 1989 when I went to Moscow to run my second marathon.

The hotel's restaurant had only two items on the menu that vegetarians could eat: boiled potatoes and sliced tomatoes. There were no other options, even though the chef attempted to conjure up other dishes to provide me additional options. It was very important to me to not compromise my way of eating. So, I was served as many boiled potatoes and sliced tomatoes that I wanted for breakfast, lunch, and dinner the entire week that I was there. I lost weight but do not recall having any ill effects running the marathon.

I no longer have feelings of being deprived. It is not depressing to eat foods that contribute to good health or move in such a way to enhance good health. There's no longer a need to give myself pity parties, because I no longer continuously must hold myself back from a lifestyle filled with unhealthiness. The bottom line is that I have no need for discipline to stay away from behaviors that contribute to my ill health. I have no need for any of that because it no longer exists in my new lifestyle. I will be able to live this way for the rest of my life.

After I crossed the lifestyle change line, family and friends indicated that they saw a positive difference because they began to understand my motivation. They finally realized and accepted the seriousness of my taking charge of my health. It seemed that they no longer were compelled to worry about my changes, like cutting my hair to a mere quarter inch to remove the need for time consuming hair prep to accommodate lunch-time runs at work; getting up before the sun to go swimming, walking, or running; no more traditional holiday meals; no need for birthday cake or any other such disease-promoting emotional eating.

The struggle to hold on to nature's ways disappeared, and I lived happily inside nature, which became as automatic as breathing. I ceased judging what others were ingesting, focusing on my own choices. I no longer wanted foods to mimic foods that did not fit according to nature's nutrition wisdom. For example, I had no tolerance for "veggie burgers," which were usually highly processed vegan junk food. I began to check in with the body around nutrition and fitness choices and make necessary adjustments if the body indicated change was needed. There was no longer a wagon to fall off. And most importantly, I felt that I had reached a personal crossroads between just existing and living a strong, gentle, kind, healthy life.

Living in this realm, I believe that I truly have something to share to make the personal world a better place for others. I became compelled to use my living to benefit others. That is the underlying reason for writing this book.

My conscious and subconscious minds have become my allies, and my body relaxed into following my new lifestyle without falter. The new me was defined by my new permanent lifestyle, not by a temporary diet-like undertaking. That's when I began to live lifestyle changes within my mind, body, and spirit. Getting to this place in my life was a real struggle, but if you can find a path to where you wish to go with no obstacles, it probably leads nowhere.

You must keep pushing harder today than you pushed yesterday to guarantee healthier tomorrows. It takes a wealth of butterfly-type patience and dandelion-type passionverance to successfully reap healthier lifestyle outcomes for the rest of your life. Remember. Using nature's principles of patience and passionverance will allow you to expertly internalize the important information presented in this section. Know that the information presented here becomes the core of the next step in the process. It is also important to note that at each step you are gradually required to be yourself in this process.

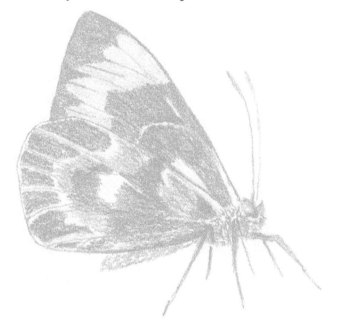

Part 3

Step Five of Nature's Six-Step Formula: Ongoing Challenges

Don't fear challenges. They often give us the opportunity to strengthen our courage, faith, and inner strength.

—Debasish Mridha

Passionverance opens the doors to step five of nature's six-step formula: ongoing challenges. You will need new challenges to prevent you from resting on your laurels. It's your mind pushing you again. It wants you to stay interested, attentive, and engrossed. It knows that you need new challenges to do so, and new challenges will keep you on the path without fail forever.

After I crossed the lifestyle change line, ongoing challenges were naturally there to greet me head-on. It was my subconscious mind that filled me full of wonder. Wondering about things pushed me to not fear challenges but to enthusiastically investigate challenges—to grab the opportunity to go further than I had ever gone before.

It worked! Wondering served to put a real jolt of momentum into identifying and working to meet ongoing challenges. Here are a few of my wonderings that came to pass over the years after I crossed the lifestyle change line.

I wondered what it might be like to run a marathon in Antarctica, on the Great Wall of China, in Moscow behind the Iron Curtain, in the desert of Egypt, and in New Zealand, as well as to run on every continent and throughout the USA. I wondered what it might be like to qualify for and run the elitist Boston Marathon, or run a 24-hour, 48-hour, 72-hour, or 144 hour ultra-marathon, without a break and on little or no sleep, or 50 miles up the side of a mountain.

Before crossing the line, I had run more than sixty marathons. I wondered what it would be like to use marathon training to train for ultra-marathons. For those unfamiliar, an ultra-marathon is any race distance beyond 26.2 miles. In the process of training for my first ultra, I trained for and ran six marathons in one year; I put all that training into running a 50K and a month later a 50 miler. I also spent lots of time wondering about taking steps to improve my nutrition. Wondering led me to gradually become a "no vegan junk food" vegan, or as my grandsons called it, a "yucky vegan." I also wondered what it might be like to become totally vegan and eat no substances from animals that have a face: cows, pigs, chickens, lambs, seafood, and all other non-plant proteins. I wondered what it would be like to eat only whole foods, complex carbohydrates, olive oil, and the lowest fat and highest fiber foods, to prepare meals that are 50 percent raw or cooked in water or at low temperatures, and even use distilled water for cooking and drinking. I wondered what it would be like to never again eat in restaurants, since it is known that there's usually unhealthy processing (overuse of salt and saturated or trans-fat) that occurs that makes unhealthy foods taste good. I wondered about the impact on the lives of my elderly neighbors who were too frail to shovel their walkways in the winter snow storms or rake the millions of leaves that fell in the fall in their yards.

These and many other challenges were realized. "I am never content with contentment," said George Sheehan. I guess with the help of my subconscious mind, I am never content with contentment as well. Like Sheehan, I am uneasy when things go easy, because to me easy is what builds comfortable ruts.

I believe that the people who make it across the lifestyle change line will automatically seek out new nutrition and fitness challenges and attack them with renewed internal strength and mind–body harmony. If they do, like me, they will find that additional trips across the lifestyle change line will keep their cells coming back stronger and stronger despite aging.

⚠ You must keep pushing harder today than you pushed yesterday to guarantee healthier tomorrows. It takes a wealth of butterfly-type patience and dandelion-type passionverance to successfully reap healthier lifestyle outcomes for the rest of your life. Remember. Using nature's principles of patience and passionverance will allow you to expertly internalize the important information presented in this section. Know that the information presented here becomes the core of the next step in the process. It is also important to note that at each step you are gradually required to be yourself in this process.

> There are so many people out there who will tell you that you can't. What you must do is turn around and say watch me.   —Unknown

Part 3

Step Six of Nature's Six-Step Formula: Healthier Outcomes

The greatest wealth is health.

— Virgil

Passionverance opens the doors to step six of nature's six-step formula: healthier outcomes. It rewards you by improving many types of health issues, including age-driven health issues. You and your doctors will notice that your blood pressure, cholesterol, blood sugar, triglycerides, heart rate, and other vital statistics are all maintaining or approaching normal limits. Most importantly, you can feel and see the difference in your energy level, stress level, and weight, as well as the great feeling you enjoy from sun up to sun up, daily. And the best part is that these are permanent changes because you have completed all six steps. You have earned the right to live each of the steps inside nature for the rest of your life.

In 2016, I participated in what I termed an "add-on" research study conducted by Johns Hopkins University research and supported by National Institutes of Health (NIH), This research was supported by the Intramural Research Program of NIH, National Institute on Aging. An add-on research study means that I was not part of the original group studied but was taken through most of data collection and related analysis that the original participants were exposed to. The name of the study was "Assessing the 'Physical Cliff': Detailed Quantification of Age-Related Differences in Daily Patterns of Physical Activity." Jennifer A. Schrack, PhD, (Jenifer Schrack, email message to me,

December 7, 2016) was the principle investigator. Her findings of my participation are summarized below:

> "Betty is about 25 percent more active than other older women attending a local wellness program (and she is an average of eight years older than the others in the group). Much of her activity takes place between 4:00 a.m. and noon … with another spike of activity in the evening between 4:00 p.m. and 8:00 p.m. Most older adults show peak activity in the morning, but few have another peak in the afternoon".
>
> —Jennifer A. Schrack, PhD.

At age seventy-seven I have an energy level that allows me to run sixty miles per week, participate in short- and long-distance races, swim more than six hours per week, practice tai chi about eight hours per week, walk about fourteen hours per week, and meditate more than seven hours per week.

⚠️ You must keep pushing harder today than you pushed yesterday to guarantee healthier tomorrows. It takes a wealth of butterfly-type patience and dandelion-type passionverance to successfully reap healthier lifestyle outcomes for the rest of your life. Remember. Using nature's principles of patience and passionverance will allow you to expertly internalize the important information presented in this Book. As a result, you will live your very own Lifestyle by Nature—forever!

Epilogue

Nature's wisdom tells us that we either live with good health or live without good health, until …

—B. H. Smith

You can begin to live a healthy life as I did when I was unhealthy and becoming unhealthier. Living a healthier life is simply living in a manner that promotes good health, not living in a manner that promotes illnesses. Unlike Hansel and Gretel, who lost their way because their bread crumbs disappeared, nature has put out six distinct crumbs that remained in place for eons, waiting for someone like me to come along, pick them up, understand and respect their worth, and follow nature's lead crumb by crumb.

Over about three decades, I followed nature's lead, albeit haphazardly at times. Hindsight helped me chronicle each nature-inspired crumb. Following her wisdom, I changed my entire lifestyle, going from unhealthy to super healthy, despite aging. And with passionverance as your secret weapon, you too can make the same permanent changes in your lifestyle and in your health.

You've already made a good beginning by reading my story. Know that your journey is just starting. All you need to do is live each of the six steps diligently. They will transform your life. Look upon them as stepping stones to a better life, where the sun forever shines upon you. Remember, the sun is always shinning, even when a cloud is in the way. Treat each challenge of your emerging new daily life as if a cloud is moving out of the way of the shining sun. Know that you will encounter peaks and valleys, which normally accompany change. Even when there seems to be no hope, know that the sun forever shines somewhere. A deeper part of you will remember that with every nutrition or movement action you either contribute to your good health or to your bad health.

Absolutely nothing out on the open market matches nature's six-step wisdom on changing lifestyles. In providing creatures the necessities of life, nature programmed into their makeup instincts that compelled them to automatically eat and move in line with nature's wisdom. Nature used the same wisdom for humans but in a different way. She provided humans with the wherewithal to access the necessities of life through what became a scientist-based process of biomimicry. It was my informal process of biomimicry that was at play when I came along and scooped up nature's nutrition and movement wisdom and applied them to my unhealthy lifestyle.

According to respected research studies that I have participated in, such as the Women's Health Initiative National Study, the Maryland University Medical School study on aging and fitness along with energy data collection headed by Johns Hopkins study on aging and energy, together with results of official labs and other medical tests, my health rivals the health of others thirty years younger.

...old habits don't have to run our lives, that our past doesn't have to become our future, and that the momentum of change ultimately leads us toward greater awareness, wisdom and peace.

—Dan Millman, *The Laws of Spirit: A Tale of Transformation*

APPENDICES

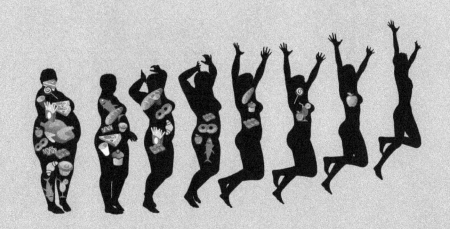

"Each step you take reveals a new horizon. You have taken the first step today. Now I challenge you to take another"

Dan Poynter

Appendix A – Nature's Nourishment

Appendix B – Alignment

Appendix C – ChiRunning

Appendix D – FYI

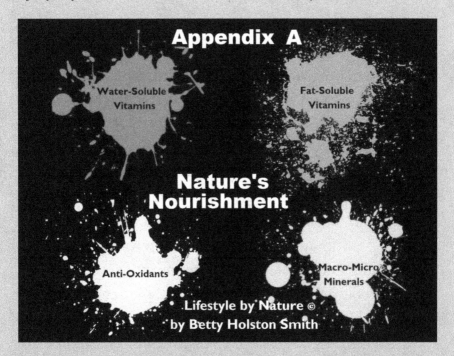

Information Sources:

Nature's Lifestyle Change System's Nourishment Charts feature the science-based nutrients from the Institute on Medicine's Food and Nutrition Board and the United States Department of Agriculture.

Instructions:

The following set of charts function as a sturdy lifeline to the best possible nutrition known by nutrition experts and provided by nature. Each chart is organized according to the type of nutrients the body needs for growth, maintenance and repair. For maximum health, the body must take in about 40 varieties to function properly according to Peter Walters and John Byt (editors) in their book entitled Christian Paths to

Health and Wellness, Second Edition. They further discuss how nutrients are grouped into overall six categories: carbohydrate, protein, lipid (fat), water, vitamins and minerals. They tell us that each category has a distinct function in the body and all categories work together to provide the body optimal health.

For simplicity, the nutrition charts below are classified according to the following four categories. The four categories together summarize the nutrients the body needs for optimal health: water-soluble vitamins, fat-soluble vitamins, antioxidants, and macro-micro minerals. For further simplicity of use, a three-column matrix is provided. The first column contains the nutrient, the second column contains the best food choices for that nutrient and the third column highlights the known health possibilities of that nutrient. For optimal health, you must ingest nutrients under each of the four categories each day.

Begin using the charts by providing yourself motivation to get on or remain on the optimal nutrition bandwagon by investigating the health possibilities in the third column. If you have health concerns, know that it is respected across many research and health experts that food can function as "your best" prevention possibilities and in certain instances, your best "non-side effect" attack for existing conditions. Next check out the best food sources in column two. The food source list can be used to establish your recipes and to make your shopping list. Make sure that you include nutrients across all four categories as you establish your recipes and shopping lists. You can vary the final serving dish from among choices such as soup, stew, separate veggie/fruit plate, or you can create your own ways of serving.

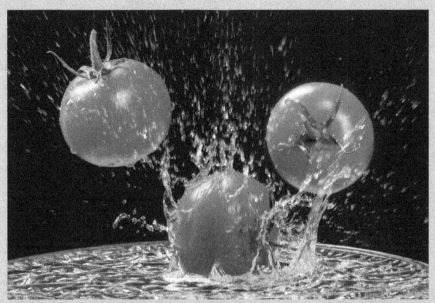

Fat-Soluble Vitamins	Examples of Best Food Sources	Health Possibilities
Vitamin A	Beta-carotene: orange and yellow fruits and vegetables, such as carrots, squash, cantaloupes, leafy greens, chia seeds	Prevents night blindness; needed for growth and cell development; maintains healthy skin, hair, nails, gums, glands, bones, and teeth; may help prevent lung cancer
Vitamin B	Made by the body when exposed to the sun; certain enriched foods	Necessary for calcium absorption; helps build and maintain strong bones and teeth
Vitamin E	Vegetable oils, nuts, and seeds	Protects fatty acids; maintains muscles and red blood cells; important antioxidant
Vitamin K	Spinach, broccoli, and other green leafy vegetables	Essential for proper blood clotting

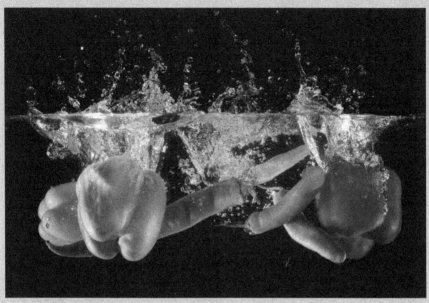

Water-Soluble Vitamins	Examples of Best Food Sources	Health Possibilities
Biotin	Soybeans, whole grains, nuts	Energy metabolism
Folate (folate acid, folacin)	Spinach and other leafy green vegetables, asparagus, avocados, legumes, oranges	Makes DNA, RNA, and red blood cells; synthesizes certain amino acids; is important for women before and after pregnancy
Niacin (vitamin B3, nicotinic acid, nicotinamide)	Legumes	Metabolizes energy; promotes normal growth; large doses lower cholesterol
Pantothenic acid (vitamin B5)	Almost all foods	Aids in energy metabolism, normalizing blood sugar levels and synthesizing antibodies, cholesterol hemoglobin, and some hormones
Riboflavin (vitamin B2)	Raw mushrooms and supplements	Essential for energy metabolism; aids adrenal function; supports normal vision and healthy skin
Thiamine (vitamin B1)	Legumes, nuts and seeds, grains	Energy metabolism; helps maintain normal digestion, appetite, and proper nerve function

Water-Soluble Vitamins	Examples of Best Food Sources	Health Possibilities
Pyridoxine, pyridoxamine, pyridoxal (vitamin B6)	Grains, bananas, leafy vegetables, potatoes, soybeans	Promotes protein metabolism, metabolism of carbohydrates, release of energy, proper nerve functions, and synthesis of red blood cells
Cobalamins (vitamin B12)	Only found in animal products and supplements	Needed to make red blood cells, DNA, RNA, and myelin (for nerve fibers)
Ascorbic acid (vitamin C)	Citrus fruits, melons, berries, peppers, broccoli, potatoes, and many other fruits and vegetables	Is a powerful antioxidant; strengthens blood vessel walls; promotes wound healing and iron absorption; helps prevent atherosclerosis; may help protect against cataracts and gout; may lower risk of certain types of cancer; supports immunity

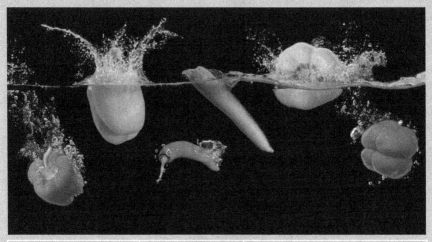

Antioxidants	Examples of Best Food Sources	Health Possibilities
Ascorbic acid (vitamin C)	Citrus fruits, melons, berries, peppers, broccoli, potatoes, many other fruits and vegetables	Is a powerful antioxidant; strengthens blood vessel walls; promotes wound healing and iron absorption; helps prevent atherosclerosis; may help protect against cataracts and gout; may lower risk of certain types of cancer; supports immunity
Vitamin E	Olive oil, nuts, seeds	May prevent heart attacks and strokes; lowers the risk of death from bladder cancer
Beta-carotene	Orange, yellow, red, and dark green fruits and vegetables, including carrots, sweet potatoes, squash, broccoli, kale, spinach, apricots, peaches, cantaloupe, watermelon	Helps prevent night blindness and age-related macular degeneration; may protect against certain types of cancer, especially lung cancer; maintains healthy skin, hair, nails, gums, glands, bones, and teeth
Lutein, zeaxanthin	Collard greens, kale, spinach, turnip greens, green peas, broccoli	Protects against cataracts and age-related macular degeneration
Lycopene	Red foods, such as tomatoes, watermelon, pink guavas	May protect against cancer, including prostate, stomach, and lung cancers

Antioxidants	Examples of Best Food Sources	Health Possibilities
Anthocyanidin	Blueberries, cherries, cranberries, blackberries, black currants, plums, red grapes	May protect against cancer and heart disease; may slow signs of aging
Hesperidin	Citrus fruits	May reduce risk of heart disease and cancer
Isoflavones	Soy, legumes, peanuts	May lower the risk of heart disease, breast cancer, and osteoporosis
Quercetin	Onions, apples, citrus fruits, tea, red wine	May help lower the risk of cancer and heart disease; may help lower high blood pressure and high cholesterol
Selenium	Brazil nuts, whole grains, onions, garlic, mushrooms, brown rice	May lower the risk of colorectal, lung, and prostate cancers; may help prevent coronary artery disease; works to protect cell membranes from oxidative damage
Coenzyme Q10	Whole grains	May help protect against heart disease

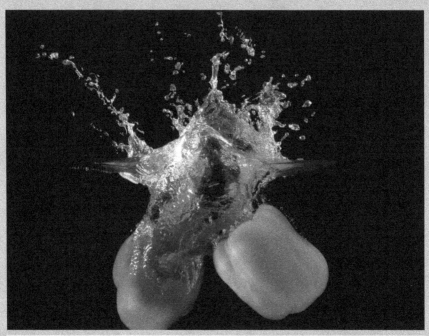

Macro-Minerals	Examples of Best Food Sources	Health Possibilities
Calcium	Dark green vegetables, tofu, sesame seeds	Builds strong bones and teeth; vital to muscle and nerve function, blood clotting, and metabolism; helps regulate blood pressure
Magnesium	Leafy green vegetables, legumes, whole grain cereals, breads, nuts	Stimulates bone growth; necessary for muscle and nerve function and metabolism; supports immunity
Phosphorus	Legumes	Helps maintain strong bones and teeth; component of some enzymes for proper metabolism

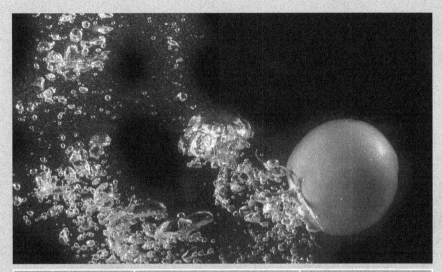

Micro-Minerals	Examples of Best Food Sources	Health Possibilities
Chromium	Whole grains, mushrooms, molasses, legumes, nuts, prunes	Works with insulin to metabolize glucose
Copper	Legumes, nuts and seeds, prunes, whole grains	Promotes iron absorption; essential to red blood cells, connective tissue, nerve fibers, and skin pigment; is a component of several enzymes
Fluoride	Tea, fluoridated water	Helps maintain strong bones and teeth
Iodine	Iodized salt, foods grown in iodized soil	Necessary to make thyroid hormones
Iron	Legumes dried fruits, whole grains, leafy greens, nuts and seeds	Needed to produce hemoglobin, which transports oxygen throughout the body
Manganese	Green and black tea, nuts, seeds, legumes, bran, leafy greens, whole grains	Component of enzymes needed for metabolism; necessary for bone and tendon formation
Molybdenum	Dark green and leafy green vegetables, whole grains, legumes, nuts	Component of enzymes needed for metabolism; instrumental in iron storage

Micro-Minerals	Examples of Best Food Sources	Health Possibilities
Selenium	Brazil nuts, whole grains, onions, garlic, mushrooms, brown rice	May lower the risk of colorectal, lung, and prostate cancers; may help prevent coronary artery disease; works to protect cell membranes from oxidative damage
Zinc	Wheat germ, nuts, legumes	Instrumental in metabolic action of enzymes; essential for growth and reproduction; supports immune function
Chloride	Table salt	With sodium, maintains fluid balance and normal cell functions
Potassium	Avocados, bananas, citrus and dried fruit, legumes, many vegetables, whole grains	With sodium, helps to maintain fluid balance; promotes proper metabolism and muscle function
Sodium	Table salt	With potassium, regulates the body's fluid balance; promotes proper nerve and muscle function

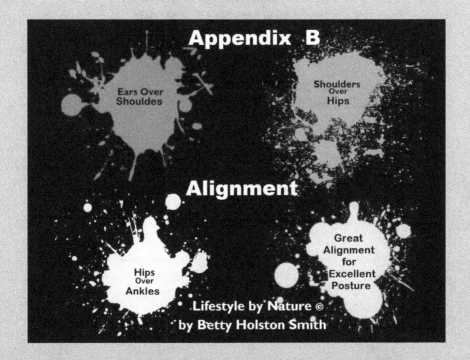

Is your posture excellent enough to serve as the foundation for all of your body movements?

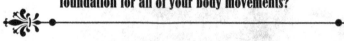

Do you know that excellent posture is all about excellent body alignment?

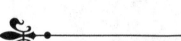

Do you know that you could easily align your body's posture by making sure that your ears, shoulder bones, hip bones and ankle bones are lined up as straight as an upright arrow?

Do you know that excellent posture along with excellent body alignment supports core strengthening?

<u>Your Bottom Line:</u>

Excellent body alignment, excellent posture and a strong core are mandatory ingredients for excellent fitness activities.

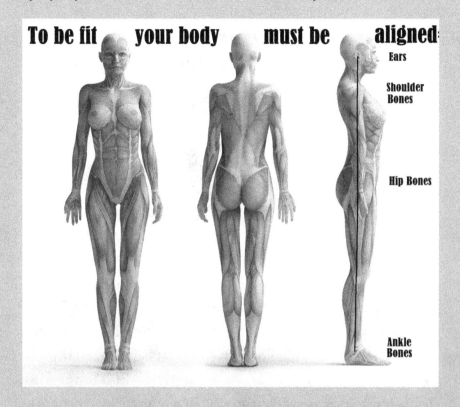

**Perfect Your Posture
to Prevent Dowager's Hump**

   Experts believe that as many as 40 percent of older adults have kyphosis, also known as dowager's hump. According to David Thomas, MD, associate professor of medicine and rehabilitation medicine at Mount Sini, dowager's hump or kyphosis is a condition that has resulted in an abnormal outward curvature of the spine in the upper back. (Thomas 2012) I believe that experts are very aware that this condition is already recruiting younger and younger people, including young children, due to poor posture alignment as electronic devices are manipulated. The downward positioning of the head used by many people is the reason the kyphosis condition will most likely ballon way beyond 40 percent for generations to come. Dr. Thomas says, "If your head juts forward, its weight pulls on the muscles in the upper back and neck, which get weak and overstretched. At the same time, the muscle in the chest get short and tight, making it difficult for you to bring your shoulders back and down. If you also have weak bones, your spine curves forward, creating a structural change."

This type of out of align posture can become severe enough to cause falls and balance issues due to a shift in the center of gravity. It can cause pain, fatigue and impede breathing and digestion because the muscles in the chest get short and tight making it difficult to squard your shoulders. Thomas says that "kyphosis is a byproduct of poor posture combining with weak muscles and bones in the upper back."

Prevention is the key because there are no recognized guidelines for its treatment. I believe that using the tactics in the following section to establish and maintain excellent posture at any age, including young children, is the most useful route for all of society to take.

Meet Your New Posture Alignment Boss

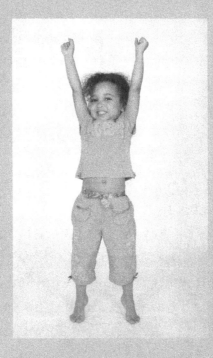

"My name is Marisol, and I am four years old. Excellent balance and alignment prepares your body to engage in injury-free movements of all types. Simply go up on your tippy toes like this; really stretch your body way, way up to the sky. At the same time, make sure that your ears are positioned over your shoulders and your chin is positioned parallel to the ground. Lower your arms and heels, but don't change your core (hips and back) positions. Next, imagine that your pelvis is a hula-hoop. Even out your pelvis by slightly lifting your pelvis up in the front. Your body is now balanced, and your posture is aligned according to nature's wisdom. Your new job is to practice this drill until your body can automatically balance and align this way 24/7."

If I can do this, *so can you!*

Your body is now all set to engage in strength, flexibility, balance, and relaxation exercises that support injury-free/energy-producing daily living activities and active movement exercises such as running, walking, skipping, soccer, basketball, swimming, dancing, horseback riding, tennis, biking, and most other active movement activities of your choice.

Now, meet the new version of you!

The "tippy toe/sky reaching" drill holds on to your S-shaped backbone as it keeps your body balanced, aligned, and upright. It positions and supports your head directly over your neck vertebra, even though you can still bend and turn your neck forward, backward, left, and right. Your pelvis, which is nearly vertical, balances your upper body directly over your strong feet and strong legs. (McCracken and Griffiths 2001)

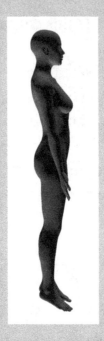

Looking at your reflection from the side, you will see that your ear, shoulder, hip, and anklebones are aligned as straight as an upright arrow. Next, level your pelvis by tipping it up in the front slightly. Your entire body is now in balanced alignment. Practice, practice, practice Marisol's "tippy toe/sky-reaching" drill constantly, until it becomes second nature.

Excellent Posture Stabilizes the Entire Body

- It stabilizes your core and vertebra, one on top of another, from your neck to your tailbone.

This movement is important because it lengthens your core, frees your diaphragm, and levels your pelvis. A lengthened core stabilizes your entire body to prevent you from leaning from your waist, putting pressure on your lower back. A freed diaphragm allows you to vigorously belly breathe. The level pelvis helps control the shape of the spine as it evens out the energy flow throughout your pelvis and lower body.

- It stabilizes your head and places it squarely on top of your core, which includes the aligned vertebra of your spine.

This movement is important because it prevents your head from tipping forward. Tipping your head forward will eventually use your smaller, weaker muscles for support, rather than nature's way of using your stronger-aligned bones and muscles.

Source: "ChiRunning" by Danny and Katherine Dreyer, 2003.

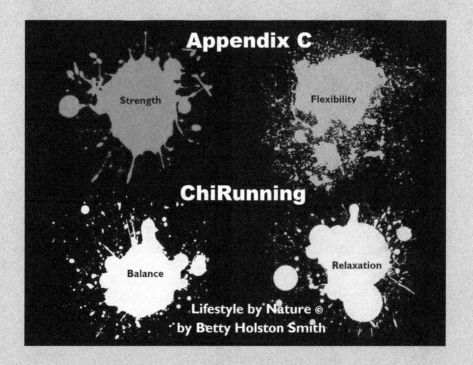

I believe stillness in motion to be moving in a manner totally in agreement with how the body was designed by nature to move. The body appears motionlessly suspended in space.

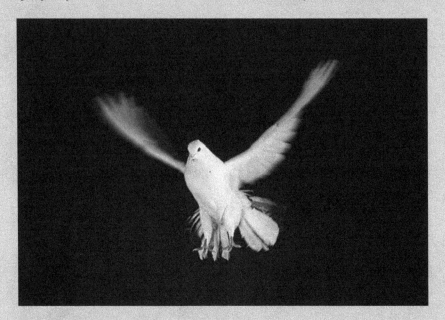

This dove is demonstrating stillness in motion technique because her core is so strong and so engaged, that it soars high above the ground, moving, but seemingly immobile. She is so graceful, so swift, so relaxed, so effortless, so like ChiRunning.

I experience ChiRunning as "stillness in motion" because my entire body appears suspended in space under the power of gravity as it moves forward. This seems so because my core is strong, straight, and silent. My head, neck, shoulders, arms, hands, and fingers are in a sleeplike, relaxed state; my hips are gracefully rotating around my spinal column as they and my legs, knees, feet, and leaning ankles are softly yielding to the recoiling of the gravity-powered forward leaning action. This state of stillness in motion can only happen when runners run in a manner totally in sync with how the body was designed by nature to run.

If you have ever witnessed dogs or horses run, or seen films of wild animals running, you have seen that it is according to this state of stillness in motion. Animals are programmed to run according to nature-bestowed instinct. The dog and three cheetahs below are demonstrating nature-bestowed instinct as they run. Each of their strong, flexible, balanced cells perform a specific job as their entire bodies automatically move forward as one unit. They are suspended in space, their feet scarcely touching down as they begin the next stride.

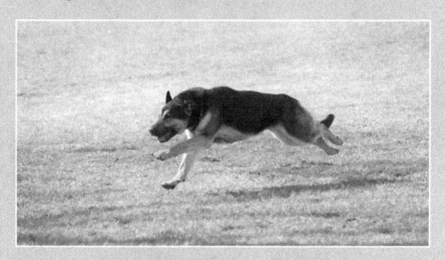

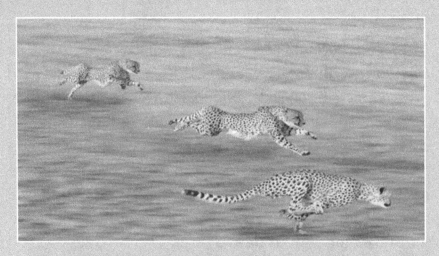

This is also true with young children. They automatically run according to nature-bestowed instinct. As such, all their body parts move forward as one unit, as each part performs the specific job assigned by nature. Young Lance below demonstrates classic ChiRunning form. His entire body appears suspended in space as he falls forward from his ankles, thereby engaging the power of gravity to propel himself forward.

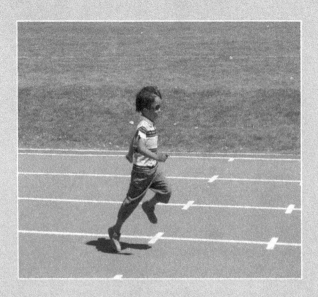

Unfortunately, the adult body can no longer run like young children because adult bodies are less flexible, less balanced, and much less relaxed. However, with passion and perseverance (or passionverance), there is a way for adults to make their way back to running like a kid again.

Danny Dreyer, the nationally ranked ultra-marathon runner and experienced tai chi practitioner, invented an approach to effortless, injury-free running called ChiRunning. ChiRunning uses the principles of tai chi to create a running form that offers increased performance with lower impact to the body.

Below is an important quote from Danny and Katherine Dreyer's first book, *ChiRunning, A Revolutionary Approach to Effortless, Injury-Free Running* (2004, page 4):

> This book presents an alternate to what we call power running. ChiRunning is based on the centuries-old principle from tai chi that states, *Less is more.* Getting back to that childhood way of running doesn't come from building bigger muscles, it comes from relaxing muscles, opening tight joints, and using gravity to do the work instead of pushing and forcing your body to move in ways that can do it harm. Most runners, especially those over thirty-five, will tell you that running can keep you in good shape, but it's hard on your body. I developed ChiRunning because I really didn't believe that pounding and injury should be a part of running. I just didn't buy it.

I must have said to myself thousands of times, "Thank you, Danny, for not buying it."

You worked hard to put all the ChiRunning, ChiWalking and ChiLiving pieces together in a way that made it possible for me to take ChiRunning to heart. I worked hard to internalize the principles of ChiRunning and can no longer run the power running way. ChiRunning taught me that my running strength comes from my center, my balance, my bones, ligaments, and tendons, not my muscles. All my muscles (except my core muscles) remain in a relaxed state. Running from my core rather than my extremities allows my muscles, tendons, and ligaments to remain in a relaxed state. Medical science agrees that it is almost impossible to hurt a relaxed muscle, tendon, or ligament. As a Chi Runner, I have run hundreds and hundreds of injury-free ultra-marathon miles with no need for recovery afterward!

As a bonus, I find that my relaxed body promotes energy recycling rather than energy draining. For example, at age seventy-four, I ran a multiday ultra-marathon on only forty minutes of sleep over the entire six days of the race. I finished the race with more energy than I had at the starting line. A comparison of my pre- and post-race blood work analyzed by my doctor showed that my oxygen-carrying red blood cells had thickened over the course of the race to provide my muscles the energy they needed. The doctor determined that my high level of health and fitness was the reason my body compensated by thickening my red blood cells.

Now at age seventy-seven, it is gratifying to continue to run sixty miles per week, all for fun, just like a kid again.

You, too, can run for fun again. Simply investigate and start ChiRunning.

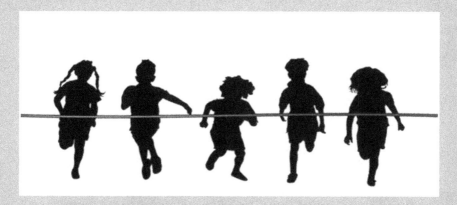

To prepare to run for fun, child-like, contact ChiLiving. com and prepare to dedicate yourself to changing how you run with less effort.

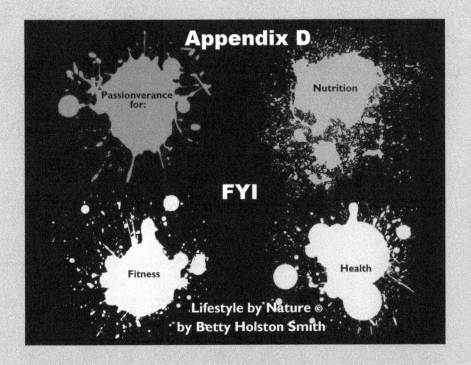

It takes constant effort to stay up to date with research outcomes. I found it critical to remain up to date, so I made sure that I could gain access to the latest information available in lay publications. That is why I have dedicated untold hours seeking out and internalizing such information for the last four decades. I've made changes in my lifestyle that have made positive differences in my ongoing levels of health and fitness. Over the years some research outcomes have changed slightly or drastically. However, I found that most research outcomes have remained stable over time. This appendix provides brief capsules of some of the more recent research outcomes in nutrition, fitness and health. The deliberate name, FYI, will hopefully encourage you to take up the banner yourself and seek out the latest information which is widely available in respected lay publications. In this way, your lifestyle will remain up to date on changes in nutrition, fitness and health practices. The sources of the information are provided if you would like to delve deeper into any topic.

NUTRITION

Tap or bottled?

Keep in mind that up to half of the bottled water produced in the U.S. comes from the tap and is then purified. And in some cases, safety standards for tap water are more rigorous than those for bottled water. People with a weakened immune system should consult their doctor to discuss whether filtered tap water or bottled water is best.

Source: Consumer Reports On Health, Volume 27, Number 7. July 2015. (Page 6)

What makes us eat too much?

Two out of three American adults—and one out of three children and teens—are overweight or obese. And it's not just here. "Since 1980, WHO estimates that the worldwide prevalence of obesity has more than doubled," noted

Margaret Chan, Director-General of the World Health Organization.

Source: Nutrition Action Health Letter (Center for Science in the Public Interest), April 2017, (Cover, Pages 3-6)

Benefits of Exercise from a Pill? Dr. Gabe Mirkin's Recommendation:

- Exercise is more effective in prolonging lives and preventing diseases than any drug on the market today. If you do not exercise, you are shortening your life.
- Exercise prevents diseases and prolongs lives through weight control, blood sugar and insulin control, skeletal and heart muscle strengthening, blood pressure control and many other benefits.
- You can prolong your endurance significantly by taking sugar in fruit and other sources during events lasting longer than 70 minutes of intense exercise.
- Eating foods or drinks with added sugars when you are not exercising can raise blood sugar to levels that can damage cells throughout your body to increases risk for obesity, diabetes and heart attacks.
- Perhaps in the future, but certainly not today, doctors may be able to prescribe a safe exercise-simulating and fat-burning drug to people who are unable to exercise because of disabilities or who are obese, diabetic or have other medical conditions that would be helped by rapid weight loss.(Mirkin 2017)

Antioxidants: Antidote to Disease.

... "These disease-preventing health-boosters are found in natural foods—especially plant foods like fruits, vegetables, nuts, seeds, and whole grains. Vitamins C and E, and the trace mineral selenium are micronutrients that act as key antioxidants in the body. . .

Avoid free-radical-forming foods such as refined carbohydrates, sugars, processed meats, red meats, deep-fried foods, and too much alcohol."

Free radicals attack your DNA or cell membranes which results in certain chronic diseases such as cancer, cardiovascular disease and diabetes.

Source: Environmental Nutrition—The Newsletter of Food, Nutrition & Health. Volume 41, Issue 3, March 2018, (Cover Page)

Is bagged salad as safe as you think?

Bags of lettuce and spinach may not be as pristine as they seem. British scientists found that during 5 days of refrigeration, traces of nutrient-rich juice released from crushed leaves in bags of salad greens nourished *Salmonella* bacteria and increased its growth by up to 280-fold compared to sterile water. The juices also enhanced the bacteria's ability to attach to the sides of the plastic bags, as well as to the leaves, as reported in *Applied and Environmental Microbiology.*

Source: Tufts University Health & Nutrition Letter, Volume 34, Number 12, February 2017. (Page 2)

Vitamin D from A to Z.

Vitamin D helps the body absorb calcium. Low levels in the blood causes more rapid bone lost.

Source: Nutrition Action Health Letter (Center for Science in the Public Interest), December 2015, (Page 7).

True or False? Fact vs fiction about the foods you eat.

- Can sugar harm your heart? Yes. Is drinking fruits and vegetables as healthy as eating them? No.
- Do whole grains lead to weight loss? Yes, if you watch the calories.
- Do beans cut cholesterol? Yes
- Is fiber the key to staying regular? Yes, but don't rely only on fiber. Also try foods with wheat bran, psyllium or prunes.
- Does green tea prevent cancer? Depends. The bottom line on green tea: Drink green tea if you like it (and if it's low in added sugar), but not to lower your risk of cancer.

Source: Nutrition Action Health Letter (Center for Science in the Public Interest). July/August 2015, Cover Story. (pages 3-6).

Cola and cancer risks

Colas and other brown soft drinks are often made with caramel color, and some contain 4-methylimidazole (4-Mel), a potential carcinogen.

Source: Consumer Reports On Health. June 2015, Volume27, Number 6, (Page 2)

On your mind (question of the month)

After I marinate meat, fish, or poultry, is it OK to use the marinade during cooking or as a sauce? No, unless you follow Department of Agriculture guidelines: Bring the marinade to a boil in a pan for 1 minute while stirring constantly. Marinade that has been in contact with raw animal protein may contain harmful bacteria.

Source: Consumer Reports On Health. September 2015, Volume 27, Number 9. (Page 12).

Reaping gains from grains.

Eating whole grains may benefit your heart and lengthen your life. Grain foods made from the hard, dry seeds of plants have been a nutritional basic for thousands of years. When you eat a whole grain, you're getting more than just the fiber from the seed's outer layer. You also get all the vitamins, minerals, good fats, enzymes, antioxidants, and phytonutrients that are stripped away when grains are processed.

Source: Harvard Medical School, Harvard Heart Letter. Volume 25, Number 8, April 2015. (cover page)

Let food be your medicine. Food has the power to nourish, protect, and heal your body.

Foods with medicinal benefits:

- Berries – rich source of phytochemicals which reduce inflammation and cancer risk.
- Broccoli – source of phytonutrients which reduce inflammation, oxidative stress, and cancer prevention.
- Cinnamon – blood sugar-balancing attributes, even with just ½ teaspoon a day.
- Cranberries – may prevent bacteria from adhering to cells inside the bladder.
- Fish – Omega-3 fatty acids in fish have anti-inflammatory properties.
- Fermented foods – supports digestive function and a healthy immune system.
- Garlic – According to the American Institute for Cancer Research, there is probable evidence that garlic and other members of the allium family reduce the risk of developing common cancers.
- Ginger and turmeric – source of anti-inflammatory and analgesic properties.
- Shiitake mushroom – anti-cancer, immune boosting and cholesterol-lowering properties.

- Nuts – helpful for cardiovascular function and healthy blood sugar and weight levels.

Source: Environmental Nutrition, Volume 17. August 2015, (Page 4)

FITNESS

Knee pain from arthritis? Try tai chi.

Could an ancient Chinese mind-body practice help with knee pain from osteoarthritis? A new Tufts study reports that tai chi produces benefits like physical therapy for osteoarthritis patients.

Source: Tufts University, Health & Nutrition Letter, November 2016, (Page 3, special report).

Take a hike

Hiking isn't just a good cardiovascular workout. It may also enhance your strength and balance while lowering your stress.

Source: Harvard Medical School, Harvard Heart Letter. Volume 27, Number 2, October 2016. (Page 5)

Exercise: medicine for the mind

Much research has shown that exercise and staying physically active in general can improve mood and help counter depression. A study in *Mayo Clinic Proceedings* in August provided some interesting evidence for this by examining what happens when active people are denied their exercise boost.

Source: University of California, Berkeley, Wellness Letter. News and Expert Advice from the School of Public Health. Volume 33, Issue 3, November 2016. (Page 6).

Intense Activity May Help Lower Your Stroke Risk

Here are reasons to step up your activity levels: Scientists have found that high-intensity exercise may protect against stroke and dementia, as well as impaired mobility and falls.

A study in the June 8, 2011, online edition of Neurology suggests that performing moderate to vigorous activity such as bicycling, swimming, jogging, hiking and playing tennis and racquetball can lower your risk of "silent" stroke.

Source: Johns Hopkins Medicine, Health After 50. Volume 23, Issue 10, December 2011. (Page 6)

Wellness made easy

Older people who stay physically active have less age-related loss of brain volume than their sedentary counterparts, according to a recent study in the *Journal of Alzheimer's Disease.* It involved 976 people over 65 who underwent periodic cognitive testing as well as MRI scans of their brains.

Source: University of California, Berkeley Wellness Letter—News and expert advice from The School of Public Health, June 2016, Volume 32, Issue 11, (page 6)

Diet, exercise may be more effective than meds for BP

Lifestyle approaches, such as reducing salt intake and saturated fat consumption, and increasing physical activity may be more effective than taking blood pressure-lowering medication, according to researcher from the University of Liverpool.

Source: Environmental Nutrition, The newsletter of food, nutrition & health, Volume 38, Issue 5, May 2015, (Cover Page)

Suffering from low back pain? Maybe you should try yoga

Two new studies offer a glimmer of hope for sufferers of chronic low back pain, from an unexpected source—yoga. The ancient physical, mental and spiritual discipline, which originated in ancient India and came to America in the 1890s, outperformed self-care for back pain in both studies.

Source: Tufts University, Health & Nutrition Letter, February 2012, Volume 29, Number 12, (Page 3)

Activity benefits go beyond weight loss

If you're looking for motivation to get up off the couch, the results of a large new European study may be just what you need to lace up those walking shoes. Even a moderate amount of exercise—the equivalent of a daily brisk 20 minute walk—was associated with significant reductions in mortality risk. Physical activity contributed to longevity independently of weight loss, and the biggest potential benefits were seen simply by going from completely sedentary to "moderately inactive".

Source: Tufts University, Health & Nutrition Letter, April 2015, (Cover Page)

Staying highly fit slows signs of aging

Older people who are highly fit, such as recreational cyclists, are physiologically more like young people than to more sedentary seniors. That's the conclusion of a new British study that sort to explore the effect of physical activity on key indicators of aging. As one scientist put it, "Being physically active makes your body function on the inside more like a young person's."

Source: Tufts University, Health & Nutrition Letter, April 2016, Volume 33, Number.2, (Page 3)

Start climbing stairs

It burns calories twice as fast as brisk walking, and it provides a great workout for your heart, lungs, legs, and arms.

Source: Harvard Medical School, Harvard Health Letter, May 2014, Volume 39, Number 7, (Page 6)

Wellness made easy

Healthy Mondays. Do you remember your New Year's resolution—to eat better and exercise more, perhaps? Or did they bite the dust a few months ago? If you've fallen off the wagon of good intentions, it's never too late to get back on, whatever the date on the calendar. And you can, of course, create new resolutions year-round.

Mondays are a good day to revisit your resolutions, according to a joint public health initiative from Johns Hopkins, Columbia, and Syracuse universities called the Monday Campaigns. That's the day of the week when most people transition back to a more structured routine— and when they are more likely to search for health-related information on the internet, start a diet or exercise program, quit smoking and make doctor's appointments. Mondays offer a "fresh "start for many people to "get their act together". According to a survey of 1,500 adults—an opportunity to celebrate a "mini-New Year 52 times a year.

Source: University of California, Berkeley Wellness Letter, News and expert advice from the School of Public Health, Volume 12, Issue 10, May 2016. (Cover Page)

Public transit commuters slimmer

Even just walking to the bus stop or train station might help commuters control their weight, according to a large British study. As expected, people who walked or biked to work had the lowest average body mass index (BMI) and percentage of body fat in the study of 150,000 middle-aged commuters. But commuters who used public transportation also had healthier body weights and compositions than those who drove.

Source: Tufts University Health & Nutrition Letter, Volume 34, Number 5, July 2016, (Page 2)

Keep active to protect your brain

Exercise may delay mental aging, preserve gray matter. Two new studies provide important evidence of how physical activity might reduce the risk of Alzheimer's disease and other forms of cognitive decline. One study reported that participants who were most active showed the least decline—the equivalent of 10 years of mental aging. In a second study, the most active older adults were found to have the largest volume of gray matter in brain regions typically affected most by Alzheimer's.

Source: Tufts University Health & Nutrition Letter, Volume 34, Number 5, July 2016, (Cover Page)

Get moving to live longer

Getting up and moving even an extra 10 minutes a day could help you live longer according to new research published in the journal *Medicine & Science in Sports & Exercise*. Unlike studies relying on self-reported activity levels, subjects wore ultra-sensitive activity trackers, called accelerometers, for seven days. About 3,000 participants, ages 50 to 79, were followed for mortality over the next eight years.

The least active people were five times more likely to die during that period than the most active participants and three times more likely than those in the middle range for activity.

Source: Tufts University Health & Nutrition Letter. Volume 34, Number 4, June 2016. (Page 6)

Even after 70, staying active pays off

Continuing to exercise as you age really can made a difference. Researchers reported in the journal *Circulation* that even people in their 70s have much lower risk of stroke and heart attack with regular moderate exercise such as walking. "When older men and women were more active, they did much better—especially with respect to heart and brain health," says Dariush Mozaffarian, MD, DrPH, dean of Tufts' Friedman School and editor-in-chief of the *Health & Nutrition Letter*. "It reassures people that even after age 75, being active can make a big difference."

Source: Tufts University Health & Nutrition Letter, Volume 34, Number 4, June 2016, (Page 6)

HEALTH

Where's the fat?

There's muscle, liver, visceral (surrounds organs) and subcutaneous (just under the skin) fat. Muscle, liver and visceral fat are more harmful than subcutaneous fat.

Source: Nutrition Action Health Letter (Center for Science in the Public Interest), April 2015, (page 4).

You are probably aware that excess weight raises your risk for cardiovascular problems and diabetes. However, something you may not know is that being overweight or obese also can significantly raise your risk for arthritis. In fact, 60 percent of people who are obese will develop osteoarthritis (OA, a subtype associated with wear and tear on the joints), with the hip and knee joints particularly susceptible.

Each pound you gain in weight translates into about four pounds of extra pressure on your knee joints.

Source: Focus on Healthy Aging, Mount Sinai School of Medicine, Volume 17, Number 10, October 2014, (cover page and page 3).

Half of heart disease deaths preventable via lifestyle choices

It is clear that lifestyle is a powerful weapon in fighting heart disease. Five preventable risk factors—high cholesterol, high blood pressure, obesity, diabetes and smoking.

Source: Environmental Nutrition, The Newsletter of Food, Nutrition & Health, Volume 38, Issue 12, December 201. (Cover Page).

We need to stop thinking about the Twinkie diet and start thinking about physiology

Says Lee Kaplan, director of the Harvard Medical School's Massachusetts Weight Center. "Exercise alters food preferences toward healthy foods. . . and healthy muscle trains the fat to burn more calories".

Source: The Washington Post, Health & Science Section, Why People Regain Weight After Dieting, January 9, 2018, Page E1

Mind your own health after the death of a partner

Taking care of yourself might be the last thing you would think about after the death of a partner. But a study published February 24, 2014, in *JAMA Internal Medicine* suggests that it may be a matter of life and death. Researchers found that a person's risk of heart attack or stroke rose in the first 30 days after a partner's death.

Harvard Medical School, Harvard Health Letter, Volume 39, Number 7, May 2014, (page 8)

From Harvard Medical School:

What you should know about skin cancer.

Follow the ABCDE rule when examining suspicious moles:

- <u>Asymmetry.</u> The shape of one half doesn't match the other.
- <u>Border.</u> A ragged or blurred edge.
- <u>Color.</u> Uneven color: it could be shades of brown, black, tan, red, white or blue.
- <u>Diameter.</u> A significant change in size resulting in a mole larger than six millimeters.
- <u>Evolving.</u> Anything changing or evolving needs to be seen by a dermatologist.

Source: Focus on Healthy Aging, Mount Sinai School of Medicine, Volume 17, Number 5, May 2015, (page 7). Reported in Weill Cornell Medical College, Women's Health/Advisor.

Fight plaque buildup in your arteries

Exercise combined with weight loss can increase "good" cholesterol and lower "bad" cholesterol. (page 3).

Learn about lower back pain

Common conditions, such as sprains and "slipped" discs, usually heal on their own. (page 4).

Use a digital fitness monitor

It tracks your exercise progress, so you can determine if you need to adjust activity levels. (page 5).

Sneak more walking into your day

Take up golf, window shop at a large mall, or visit a walking-only destination such as a museum or botanical garden. (page 5).

Harvard Medical School, Harvard Health Letter. Volume 39, Number 9, July 2014

Walking outside barefoot may help your health, research shows

This was the headline in a recent Washington Post Wellness section article by Carrie Dannett, a registered dietitian, nutritionist and owner of Nutrition by Carrie. Dannett began her piece by stating, in part, the importance of spending time in nature and how for years "Researchers have been detailing how people who live near green spaces – parks, greenbelts, three-lined streets, rural landscapes—have better physical and mental health."

Dannett goes on to discuss a process of walking barefoot in nature is called grounding (also called earthing). "The idea behind grounding is humans evolved in contact with the Earth's electric charge but lost that connection because of innovations such as buildings and shoes. Grounding advocates say this disconnect might be contributing to chronic disease.

What's more Dannett continues, "Contact with the Earth's surface could provide antioxidants and regulate our nervous system and internal clock." She advises us all to try it out. Interested or curious people can learn more on the Earthing Institute website: locallliving@washpost.com

Source: The Washington Post – Thursday, July 12, 2018

Move of the month: pelvic tilt.

Relieve back pain by strengthening abdominal muscles. Lie on your back with your arms at your sides, knees bent, feet flat on the floor and hip-with apart. Exhale as you tighten your abdominal muscles as if pulling your navel toward your spine, and slightly tilt your pelvis, flattening your lower back on the floor. Hold. Return to the starting position. Repeat eight to ten times.

Harvard Medical School, Harvard Health Letter, Volume 39, Number 9, July 2014, (page 4).

Make a habit of standing more and sitting less.

Even if you get plenty of exercise, being sedentary most of the day is a bad idea.

Source: Harvard Medical School, Harvard Health Letter,Volume 25, Number 9, May 2015, (page 4).

Give your neck a break.

Don't hold it in a bent position for more than 10 minutes, whether you're reading or looking at a smartphone or computer.

Source: Harvard Medical School, Harvard Health Letter, Volume 39, Number 7, May 2014, (page 4).

Brain-training games

Last fall, more than 60 neuroscientists and other experts signed a letter which noted, "No studies have demonstrated that playing brain games cures or prevents Alzheimer's disease or other forms of dementia." Your best bet for fending off memory and thinking problems may be a combination of regular exercise, a healthy diet, sound sleep and engaging in new activities, such as studying another language, taking dance lessons, or learning to play a new instrument.

Source: Consumer Reports on Health, The truth about what's good for you. Volume 27, Issue 8, August 2015, (Page 12)

How to stay hydrated

Most people drink when they feel thirsty, which seems to work. But as we age, the sense of thirst is less acute, and the body is less able to conserve water. Some drugs and medical conditions also increase urine output. All increases the risk of dehydration, which can be life-threatening. The color of your urine can indicate if you're well-hydrated, says Marvin M. Lipman, M.D., Consumer Reports' chief medical adviser. If it's clear you are drinking too much. If it's concentrated and dark yellow, you are drinking too little. It should be in between.

Source: Consumer Reports on Health, The truth about what's good for you. Volume 27, Number 7, July 2015, (Page 7).

Too much TV time?

When researchers in Japan tracked more than 86,000 people for 18 years, they found that those who watched TV for 5 hours or longer per day had double the risk of blood clots compared with those who watched less than 2 ½ hours daily.

Reported in Consumer Reports on Health, The truth about what's good for you. Volume 27, Number 12, December 2015, (Page 3)

Source: Presented Aug. 29, 2015, at the European Society of Cardiology 2015 Congress.

The downside of too much sitting

Standing up more throughout the day may help you dodge heart disease and live longer.

Source: Harvard Medical School, Harvard Heart Letter, Volume 25, Number 9, May 2015, (Page 4).

Produce for stronger bones.

Potassium, found in many fruits and veggies, can help reduce the risk of brittle bones and fractures by slowing the loss of calcium from bone, according to a recent review of 14 studies by researchers at England's University of Surrey. Most Americans get just half of the recommended 4,700 milligrams of dietary potassium per day. Boost your intake of high potassium produce, such as baked potatoes with the skin on (800 milligrams in a medium potato), broccoli (460 per cup), and banana (450 in a medium one).

Reported in Consumer Reports on Health, The truth about what's good for you. Volume 27, Number 5, May 2015, (Page 3). Source: Osteoporosis International, Jan 9, 2015.

Arthritis warning sign

Research on 4,673 Americans who had knee arthritis or were at risk for it indicates that pain while going up or down stairs may be the first sign of osteoarthritis in the knees.

Reported in Consumer Reports On Health, The truth about what's good for you. Volume 27, Number 5, May 2015, (Page 3)

Source: Arthritis Care & Research, January 2015.

New Heart Attack Prevention Guidelines

By Gabe Mirkin, MD
November 2018

(Re-printed with permission from Dr. Gabe Mirkin)

On November 10, 2018, heart specialists presented the latest recommendations for preventing heart attacks from the American College of Cardiology and the American Heart Association at the AHA's 2018 Scientific Sessions in Chicago (*J of the Am Coll of Card* and the AHA journal, *Circulation*, November 2018). Specifically, they recommend that doctors:

- Treat all of their patients with recommendations for heart-attack-preventing lifestyle changes, and
- Treat all patients with significant heart attack risk factors with medications that lower blood levels of the bad LDL cholesterol.

Statins have been recommended for many years, but the heart specialists also recommend the use of ezetimibe (brand name Zetia), which is now available inexpensively as a generic drug. Ezetimibe reduces the amount of cholesterol absorbed in the small intestines. They also recommend use of PCSK9 inhibitors that block a process that prevents the liver from removing LDL from the bloodstream. The price of one brand of these PCSK9 inhibitors has been reduced from $14,000 per year, but it still costs nearly $6,000 per year.

The new guidelines recommend that:

- People under age 75 who have a lot of plaques in their arteries should be given "high-intensity" statin treatment to reduce LDL by at least 50 percent.
- Middle-aged diabetics (aged 40-75) should be given "moderate intensity" statin therapy.
- People with a known history of heart disease should be given statins plus ezetimibe. If LDL is not below 70, PCSK9 inhibitors should be added.
- People with genetic (familial) high cholesterol should be treated to get their LDL cholesterol below 100 with statins, and if necessary, ezetimibe and PCSK9 inhibitors.
- All diabetics should be treated with intensive lifestyle changes

Basis for the New Guidelines

Heart attacks are caused by plaques breaking off from the inner lining of arteries. These new guidelines are based on research showing that arteriosclerotic plaques start to form at LDL cholesterol levels at 50 to 60 mg/dL and plaques do not start to regress until LDL levels drop below 50 (*J of the Am Coll of Cardiol*, Dec 19, 2017;70:2979-2991). The cardiologists now consider LDL levels greater than 160 mg/dl to be very high, and they recommend treating high risk patients to achieve LDL levels below 70 mg/dl.

Heart Attack Risk Factors

- high systolic blood pressure: >120 at bedtime
- high cholesterol: non-HDL cholesterol >130 mg/dL (below 3.4 mmol/L)
- high triglycerides: >150
- high blood sugar: >140 mg/dl one hour after meals
- high HBA1C: >5.7 (diabetes)
- small LDL particle size (an indicator of diabetes)
- high CRP: >1 (a measure of inflammation)
- high Lp(a): >130 (a genetic clotting condition)
- high homocysteine: >10
- abdominal obesity: pinch 3" or more of skin and fat near belly button
- family history of heart attacks
- having autoimmune or inflammatory conditions such as psoriasis, HIV, rheumatoid arthritis, lupus or kidney disease, which increases risk for heart disease

Lifestyle factors that increase risk of heart disease include:

- smoking
- taking more than one alcoholic drink a day
- not exercising for 30 minutes at least five times a week
- not eating lots of plants (vegetables, fruits, beans, nuts and so forth)
- eating a lot of sugar-added foods, sugared drinks, red meat, processed meat or fried foods

Coronary Artery Calcium Score

In addition to tests for the risk factors listed above, doctors may order a special CT X ray of the heart arteries that can tell if a person has lots of plaques in his heart arteries and if the plaques are likely to break off to cause heart attacks. Scores greater than 100 are associated with a slightly increased risk and scores greater than 500 show significant increased risk. A radiologist can predict if a plaque is stable or unstable (likely to break off to cause a heart attack). Plaques that have breaks in the calcium lining the inner plaque and are full of fat are the ones most likely to break off to cause heart attacks.

Endurance athletes should be warned that they can have high calcium scores even though they may be at low risk for heart attacks. Over time, endurance exercise can increase the size of coronary arteries and since area equals the square of the radius, doubling the size of an artery quadruples the calcium score. These athletes are likely to have large amounts of plaque but the arteries will still be open wide enough for plenty of blood to circulate.

A calcium score X ray exposes a person to radiation, so discuss the pros and cons of this test with your doctor.

Dr, Mirkin's Recommendations

Today, more than one third of North Americans are at high risk for heart attacks because of unhealthful lifestyles. Everyone should follow the guidelines for healthful living from an early age to help prevent heart attacks as well as strokes, dementia, diabetes and many other diseases. Check with your doctor.

Glossary

Automatic negative thoughts (ANT): A term that describes negative thoughts in the mind–body field. As the term implies, negative thoughts can happen so habitually that one does not realize that such thoughts seriously minimize chances of achieving even the simplest challenge.

Biomimicry: A term coined in the 1950s by American biophysicist Otto Schmitt. It is the human copying of nature's time-tested wisdom to make life much better by making it simpler and more sustainable for humans and the environment here on earth. Inventors over many years have copied nature's wisdom in attempts to make life better for us.

ChiRunning: A method of running using the power of gravity rather than muscle power to propel forward motion.

ChiWalking: A method of walking using the power of gravity rather than muscle power to propel forward motion.

Eighth wonder of the natural world. Akin to the list of the seven wonders of the ancient world, in 1997 CNN created a list of the seven wonders of the natural world. The CNN editors were so enthralled with the brilliance and the massive natural beauty created by nature that they formulated the natural list to celebrate nature's incredible genius.

Nature, the architect of nature's six-step formula, began prepping me to uncover its existence back in the early 1970s. It took until the 1990s to gradually live and prove the worth of all six steps.

The eighth wonder of the natural world is nature's lifestyle change system and its six-step formula. I saw nature's six-step formula as a worthy addition to CNN's list because, in my view, it is one of nature's wonders. Without knowledge, permission or participation of CNN, I informally added nature's six-step formula to CNN's list as the eighth wonder of the natural world.

Emotional nutrition: Eating to satisfy desire, taste and convenience at the expense of eating to satisfy good nutrition.

Emotional fitness: Moving to satisfy desire, feelings and convenience at the expense of moving to reap health benefits.

Nature's golden standard: The strong, flexible, balanced, and relaxed dandelion.

Nature's secret ingredient: Nature's secret ingredient is passion and perseverance banded together called passionverance.

Nature's six-step formula:

Step one is internal strength: The subconscious strength of will that furthers the crusade to achieve lifestyle challenges.

Step two is mind–body harmony: The coordination of the work between the mind and the body as they team up to further the crusade to achieve lifestyle challenges.

Step three is nutrition and movement harmony: The coordination of the work between nutrition and movement as they team up to further the crusade to achieve lifestyle challenges.

Step four is the lifestyle change line: The achievement after taking steps one to three to heart. Crossing the line means that your lifestyle-change struggles disappear as you live your healthier life.

Step five is ongoing challenges: Important to remaining interested, attentive, and engrossed in your new lifestyle. Ongoing challenges do not allow you to rest on your laurels.

Step six is healthier outcomes: The health rewards that you will enjoy for the rest of your life.

One Breath Focus: The mind follows the path the breath takes on inhale and exhale.

One Swallow, One Breath: Remaining in the present moment when eating and moving.

Passionverance: A term that summarizes the power of passion with the energy of perseverance. It is the concentrated combination of having true love for something and at the same time having the staying power to achieve it.

Positive Linkups (PLUS): Changing the mindset from negative to positive through establishing and maintaining excellent posture and carrying out the One Breath Focus breathing technique.

Qualities of success principles: These principles are among the qualities that successful people are known to routinely have or work toward: ego management, open to change, risk taking, thriving on pressure, and goal-oriented.

Senescent Cells: As you age, some cells in your body become senescent cells. Senescent cells are abnormal cells. They try to live forever, stop producing new cells and they lose their ability to perform normal functions. Most senescent cells are destroyed by your immune system. Those not destroyed can become cancerous. An anti-inflammatory lifestyle destroys senescent cells. For additional information, call up drmirkin.com and search senescent cells.

Ultra-marathon: Any running or walking distance beyond the 26.2-mile marathon distance.

YUCK: This stands for yams, unsaturated fats, chia seeds, and kale. YUCK represents a way of eating which is vegan and organic and uses unprocessed, low-fat, and high-fiber foods.

References

Andrews, Roy, 1951, *Nature's Ways: How Nature Takes Care of its Own. New York:* Avenel Books

Beilock, Sian, 2010, *Choke: What the Secrets of the Brain Reveal about Getting It Right When You Have To.* New York: Free Press, A Division of Simon & Schuster, Inc.

Beilock, Sian, 2015. *How the Body Knows Its Mind: The Surprising Power of Physical Environment to Influence How You Think and Feel.* New York: Atria Books.

Bellis, Mary, Updated April 1, 2016. *Who Invented Velco?* Thought Co. https://www.thoughtco.com/who-invented-velcro-4019660

Chaudhary, Kulreet, MD. 2016. *Prime. New York, New York: Harmony Books*

Dreyer, Danny and Dreyer Katherine 2004. *ChiRunning: A Revolutionary Approach to Effortless, Injury-Free Running* New York, New York, Fireside Books.

Lodge, Henry, MD & Crowley, Christopher, 2007, *Younger Next Year.* New York, New York. Workman Publishing Company, Inc.

Lodge, Henry, MD, March 18, 2007, *You Can Stop "Normal" Aging:* The Washington Post, Parade Magazine:

Mayo Clinic, *Exercise: 7 Benefits of Regular Physical Activity.* <u>http://www.mayoclinic.org/healthy-lifestyle/</u> <u>fitness/in-depth/exercise/art-20048389/</u> Accessed October 15, 2016.

Mayo Clinic Prevent Back Pain with Excellent Posture" n.d. Accessed October 2015. https://www.mayoclinic.org/ healthy-lifestyle/adult-health/multimedia/back-pain/sls-20076817 Image by Dreamstime.com.

MCCracken, Thomas, (General Editor) Weller, Richard (Contributing Editor), Glenn, Jim (Senior Writer), 2011, *Anatographica: A Fantastic Three-Dimensional Journey into the Body, How the Amazing Human Machine Works— From the cellular Level to Complete Systems.* China, BCL Press.

McCracken,Thomas (General Editor) and Griffiths, Martain (Contributing Editor) 2001, *Wall Chart of Human Anatomy, 3D Full-Body Images and Detailed System Charts. China, Barnes and Noble Books.*

Mirkin, Gabe, MD May 25, 2014. <u>http://www.drmirkin.</u> <u>com/nutrition/eat-your-greens-beans-and-nuts.html</u>.

Mirkin, Gabe, MD May 2007. *New Data on Meat.* <u>http://</u> <u>www.drmirkin.com/nutrition/new-data-on-meat.html</u>.

Mirkin, Gabe MD May 2017. *Benefits of Exercise From a Pill?* http://www.drmirkin.com/fitness/benefits-of-exercise-from-a-pill.html

Mirkin, Gabe MD October 2018, Healthy Aging and Senescent Cells, http://drmirkin.com/Fitnessand Health e-zine. Drmirkin.com.

Mure, Nancy S. n.d. "Obesity is not a disease" Accessed August 3, 2005" https://www.goodreads.com/quotes/7512806-obesity-is-not-a-disease-it-is-a-lifestyle-affliction

National Institutes of Health (*NIH Medline Plus, 2008*). https://medlineplus.gov/magazine/issues/winter08/articles/winter08pg4.html. Accessed August 2, 2017).

National Geographic Headquarters in Washington, D.C., In a speech, Richard Louv explains that the term nature-deficit disorder is not clinically recognized, but argues that nature-deficit disorder affects "health, spiritual well-being, and many other areas, including [people's] ability to feel ultimately alive." Accessed January 2, 2014. http://news.nationalgeographic.com/news/2013/06/130623-richard-louv-national-deficit-disorder-health-environment.html.

Nightingdale, Earl n.d.: "Whatever we plant in our subconscious mind and nourish with repetition and emotion will one day become our reality" Accessed February 15, 2008. https://www.goodreads.com/author/quotes/140743. Earl Nightingale.

Parade Magazine, Washington Post, March 18, 2007, page 6.

Pelletier, Kenneth, 1995, *Sound Mind, Sound Body: A New Model for Lifelong Health.* New York: Fireside Books Rodale Press, Emmaus, PA.

President's Council on Fitness,Sports & Nutrition n.d. https://search.hhs.gov/search?q=why+are+bone+ strengthening+exercise+ important?&HHS=Search&site =HHS &entqr=3&ud=1&sort=date:D:L:d1&output =x m l _n o _d t d & i e = U T F - 8 & o e = U T F - 8&lr=lang_en&client=HHS&proxystylesheet= fitness_drupal&filter=0&ulang=en&&access= p&entqrm=3&entsp=a__ hhsgov_policy&wc=200&wc _mc=1&start=10

Sheehan, George MD, 1989, *Personal Best:The Foremost Philosopher of Fitness Shares Techniques and Tactics for Success and Self-Liberation*

Thomas, David MD, 2012, *Perfect Your Posture to Help Prevent Dowager's Hump.* Focus on Healthy Aging, Mount Sinai School of Medicine, Volume 15, Number 7. Tufts Health Nutrition Letter, May 2007.

Walters, Peter, Byl, John 2013, *Christian Paths to Health and Wellness*, 2nd Edition, Human Kinetics Publishers, Champaign, Il.

Bibliography

Alzheimer's Foundation of America. Alzheimer's Prevention. Accessed September 18, 2013.

American Geriatrics Society. Accessed September 18, 2013.

Armstrong S et al. 2009. "Social Connectedness, Self-Esteem, and Depression Symptomatology Among Collegiate Athletes Versus Nonathletes." *Journal of American College Health* 57:521–526.

Berman, M.G, J Jonides, and S Kaplan. 2008. "The Cognitive Benefits of Interacting with Nature." *Psychological Science* 19(12):1207–1212.

Bowler, DE, LM Buyung-Ali, TM Knight, and AS Pullin. 2010. "A Systematic Review of Evidence for the Added Benefits to Health of Exposure to Natural Environments." *BMC Public Health* 10:456.

Bringslimark, T, G Patil, T Hartig. 2008. "The Association Between Indoor Plants, Stress, Productivity and Sick Leave in Office Workers." *Acta Horticulturae* 775:117.

Centers for Disease Control and Prevention. 2013. "The State of Aging and Health in America 2013. Accessed

September 18, 2013. https://www.cdc.gov/aging/pdf/state-aging-health-in-america-2013.pdf.

Centers for Disease Control and Prevention. 2015. "Physical Activity and Health." http://www.cdc.gov/physicalactivity/everyone/health/index.html. Accessed September 6, 2016.

Cervinka, R, K Röderer, and E Hefler. 2012. "Are Nature Lovers Happy? On Various Indicators of Well-Being and Connectedness with Nature." *Journal of Health Psychology* 17(3):379–388.

Cleveland Clinic Foundation.

Coley, R, FE Kuo, and WC Sullivan. 1997. "Where Does Community Grow? The Social Context Created by Nature in Urban Public Housing." *Environment and Behavior* 29(4):468.

Devries, S. 2003. "Natural Environments—Healthy Environments? An Exploratory Analysis of the Relationship Between Greenspace and Health." *Environment and Planning* 35(10):1717.

Diette, GB, N Lechtzin, E Haponik, A Devrotes, and HR Rubin. 2003. "Distraction Therapy with Nature Sights and Sounds Reduces Pain During Flexible Bronchoscopy: A Complementary Approach to Routine Analgesia." *Chest* 123(3):941–948.

Fredrickson, BL, MM Tugade, CE Waugh, GR Larkin. 2003. "What Good Are Positive Emotions in Crises? A Prospective Study of Resilience and Emotions Following the Terrorist Attacks on the United States on September 11th, 2001." *Journal of Personality and Social Psychology* 84(2):365–376.

Gilbert, S, EK Kelloway. 2014. "Positive Psychology and the Healthy Workplace." In *Workplace Well-Being: How to Build Psychologically Healthy Workplaces,* edited by A Day, EK Kelloway, and JJ Hurrell, Jr., 50–71. New York: Wiley-Blackwell.

Goleman, D. 1987. "Research Affirms Power of Positive Thinking." *New York Times,* February 3. Accessed August 1, 2017. http://www.nytimes.com/1987/02/03/science/research-affirms-power-of-positive-thinking.html?pagewanted=all.

Goode, E. 2003. "Power of Positive Thinking May Have a Health Benefit, Study Says." *New York Times,* September 2. Accessed August 1, 2017. http://www.nytimes.com/2003/09/02/health/power-of-positive-thinking-may-have-a-health-benefit-study-says.html.

Hartig, T. 1991. "Restorative Effects of Natural Environment Experiences." *Environment and Behavior* 23:3.

Jensen-Campbell, LA, JM Knack, HL Gomez. 2010. "The Psychology of Nice People." *Social and Personality Psychology Compass* 4(11);1042–1056.

Kim, T. 2010. "Human Brain Activation in Response to Visual Stimulation with Rural and Urban Scenery Pictures: A Functional Magnetic Resonance Imaging Study." *Science of the Total Environment* 408(12):2600.

Kuo, F. 2001. "Aggression and Violence in the Inner City: Effects of Environment Via Mental Fatigue." *Environment and Behavior* 33(4):543.

Langens, TA, S Morth. 2003. "Repressive Coping and the Use of Passive and Active Coping Strategies." *Personality and Individual Differences* 35(2):461–473.

Largo-Wight, E, WW Chen, V Dodd, and R Weiler. 2011. "Healthy Workplaces: The Effects of Nature Contact at Work on Employee Stress and Health." *Public Health Reports* 126 Suppl 1:124–130.

Laskowski ER (expert opinion). Mayo Clinic, Rochester, Minn. September 6, 2016.

Lodge, HS, MD, C Crowley, MD. 2007. *Younger Next Year.* New York: Workman Publishing Company.

Lohr, V. 2007. "Benefits of Nature: What We Are Learning About Why People Respond to Nature." *Journal of Physiological Anthropology* 26(2):83.

Magee, E, MPH, RD. 2014. 2009. "How Food Affects Your Moods." Accessed August 1, 2017. http://www.webmd.com/food-recipes/how-food-affects-your-moods.

Marcus, C, and M Barnes, eds. 1999. *Healing Gardens: Therapeutic Benefits and Design Recommendations*. New York: John Wiley and Sons.

Mayer, FS, CM Frantz, E Bruehlman-Senecal, and K Dolliver. 2009. "Why Is Nature Beneficial?" *Environment and Behavior* 41(5):607–643.

Mayo Clinic Staff. 2014. "Water: How Much Should You Drink Every Day?" Accessed August 1, 2017.http://www.mayoclinic.org/healthy-lifestyle/nutrition-and-healthy-eating/in-depth/water/art-20044256.

Mayo Clinic Staff. 2017. "Positive Thinking: Stop Negative Self-Talk to Reduce Stress." Accessed August 1, 2017. http://www.mayoclinic.com/health/positive-thinking/SR00009.

McCracken, TO, ed. 2011. *Anatographica: A Fantastic Three-Dimensional Journey into the Body*. New York: BCL Press.

Mind Organization. 2007. *Ecotherapy: The Green Agenda for Mental Health*. UK: Mind Publications.

Mitchell, R, and F Popham. 2008. "Effect of Exposure to Natural Environment on Health Inequalities: An Observational Population Study." *Lancet* 372(9650):1655–1660.

Moore SC et al. 2016. "Association of Leisure-Time Physical Activity with Risk of 26 Types of Cancer in 1.44 Million Adults." *JAMA Internal Medicine* 176:816–825.

NASA. "Plants Clean Air and Water for Indoor Environments." Accessed May 11, 2013. http://spinoff.nasa.gov/Spinoff2007/ps_3.html.

National Institutes of Health. Winter 2007. "7 Steps to Aging Well." *Medline Plus* 2(1):14-16.

National Institutes of Health. Winter 2008. "Emotions and Health." *Medline Plus* 3(1):4.

Pelletier, K, MD. 2002. "Mind as Healer, Mind as Slayer: Mind Body Medicine Comes of Age." *Advances in Mind–Body Medicine* 18:4–15.

Peterson DM. 2017. http://www.uptodate.com/contents/the-benefits-and-risks-of-exercise?source=search_result&search=Overview+of+the+benefits+and+risks+of+exercise.&selectedTitle=1~150.Accessed August 1, 2017.

Proyer, RT. 2014. "A Psycho-Linguistic Approach for Studying Adult Playfulness: A Replication and Extension Toward Relations with Humor." *Journal of Psychology* 148(6):717–735.

Schwartz, T. 2003. "Positive Thinking." *Chronicle Magazine*. Accessed August 1, 2017. http://www.lclark.edu/live/news/18064-positive-thinking.

Segerstrom, S., and S Sephton. 2010. "Optimistic Expectancies and Cell-Mediated Immunity: The Role of Positive Affect." *Psychological Science* 21(3):448–555.

Selub, E, and A Logan. 2012. *Your Brain on Nature: The Science of Nature's Influence on Your Health, Happiness and Vitality*. Mississauga, Ontario: Wiley.

Shepley, M, R Gerbi, A Watson, and S Imgrund. "Patient and Staff Environments: The Impact of Daylight and Windows on ICU Patients and Staff." *World Health Design*. Accessed August 1, 2017. http://www.worldhealthdesign.com/Patient-and-staff-environments.aspx.

U.S. Department of Health and Human Services. "Physical Activity Guidelines for Americans." http://www.health.gov/paguidelines/guidelines/default.aspx. Accessed September 6, 2016.

U.S. Department of Health and Human Services. 2017. "Get Enough Sleep." Accessed August 1, 2017.

http://healthfinder.gov/HealthTopics/Category/everyday-healthy-living/mental-health-and-relationship/get-enough-sleep.

Ulrich, RS, RF Simons, BD Losito, E Fiorito, MA Miles, and M Zelson. 1991. "Stress Recovery During Exposure to Natural and Urban Environments." *Journal of Environmental Psychology* 11(3):201–230.

van der Berg, A. 2010. "Green Space as a Buffer Between Stressful Life Events and Health." *Social Science & Medicine* 70(8):1203–1210.

WebMD. 2016. "Exercise and Depression." Accessed August 1, 2017. http://www.webmd.com/depression/guide/exercise-depression.

Weinstein, N. 2009. "Can Nature Make Us More Caring? Effects of Immersion in Nature on Intrinsic Aspirations and Generosity." *Personality and Social Psychology Bulletin* 35:1315.

About the Author

Betty Holston Smith grew up in the 1940s and 1950s in Chevy Chase, Maryland, amidst nature-rich virgin woods, in a family whose parents imparted passion for learning to all six of their children. Betty's passion for learning manifested as wondering about everything in nature's virgin woods and beyond.

As a child, Smith devised an investigatory routine that helped to satisfy her passion. First, she played up her passion for wondering by simply wondering—about most things. She then copiously scrutinized the situation her wondering focused on at the time. Next, she dissected the focused situation and extracted its essential parts. And finally, she satisfied her wondering of the focused situation by becoming a copycat, attempting to replicate or imitate nature's wisdom.

For example, as a child Smith wondered if she could successfully transplant one of nature's colorful wildflower gardens from the woods into her own yard. She wondered what it might be like to shriek in fun like the white kids in the deep end of the county's segregated swimming pool. She wondered what it would take to continue her education through the terminal degree as a part-time student and a full-time wife, mother, and employee. She wondered what it would take to give up junk food, lose weight, become active, and stop smoking.

In her thirties, Smith took five years of swimming lessons and did indeed shriek in fun in the deep end. As a part-time student, she completed three degrees, which took thirty-two years beyond high school. She trashed diets in favor of using the biomimicry process of copying nature's lifestyle change wisdom to maintain an eighty-pound weight lost over forty-four years and becoming a non-smoking, vegan-eating, ultra-marathon runner. She did all of this and much more by living nature's Lifestyle Change System's six-step formula.

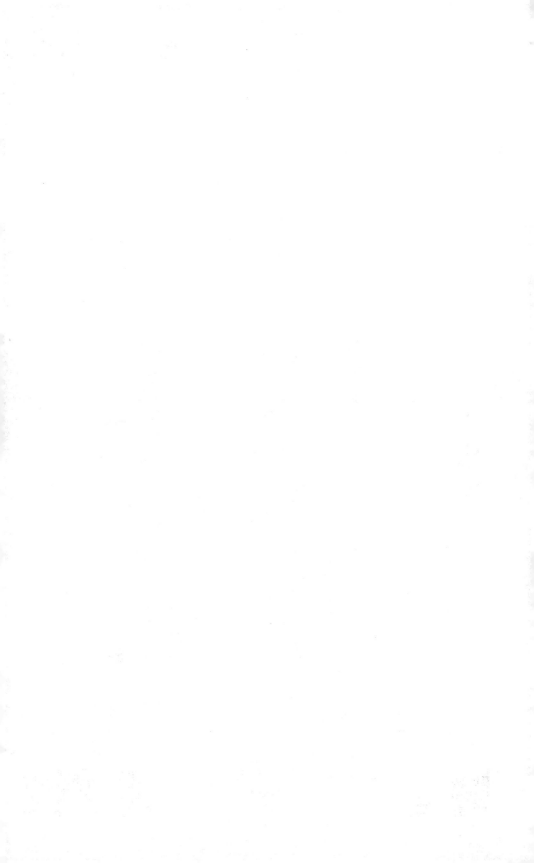

CPSIA information can be obtained
at www.ICGtesting.com
Printed in the USA
LVHW030317240920
666980LV00001B/185

9 781546 216216